MAXIMUM
FAT LOSS

MAXIMUM FAT LOSS

TED BROER

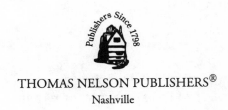

THOMAS NELSON PUBLISHERS®

Nashville

Published in Nashville, Tennessee, by Thomas Nelson, Inc.

Scripture quotations are from THE NEW KING JAMES VERSION. Copyright © 1979, 1980, 1982, Thomas Nelson, Inc., Publishers.

Library of Congress Cataloging-in-Publication Data

Broer, Ted.
    Maximum fat loss : you don't have a weight problem! It's much simpler than that / Ted Broer.
      p. cm.
    ISBN 0-7852-6711-5
    1. Weight loss. I. Title.
    RM222.2.B7815 2001
    613.7—dc21

                                         00-066839
                                            CIP

Printed in the United States of America

1 2 3 4 5 6 7 8 9 BVG 05 04 03 02 01

CONTENTS

Introduction

FAT . . . AND GETTING FATTER AND SICKER

Americans are the fattest people on earth. No nation on earth is more preoccupied with dieting than the United States. Even so, there are no people on earth who are as fat as we are.

A third of us are at least 20 percent overweight and about three-quarters of us are heavier than our optimal weight. We've gained a whopping twelve pounds per person, on the average, in just the last decade.[1]

At least that's what the statisticians tell us. I believe these figures are low. Just watch the people walk by on a beach or in a busy airport and mentally calculate the percentage of people who are carrying around excess fat. I think you'll agree with me that the percentage is about 50 to 60 percent. Sadly, about a third of our children are also obese.

One of the amazing facts to me is that given the mass media onslaught against fat and the many exercise programs available to the public, we don't seem to care that we are fat. At least we don't seem to care enough to do anything about it. All around me I see signs that people celebrate the fact that they are overweight, declaring that "big is beautiful" and advocating "fat acceptance." There's even a National Association for the Advancement of Fat Acceptance, which declares that an obsession with thinness is basically a prejudice against fat people.

The science of weight management, however, says otherwise. *Obesity is a serious physical ailment.*

In my work with thousands of clients through the years, helping them to implement health and fitness programs, I have found that few people really know just how harmful their excess fat can be. Let me share with you some scientifically based facts.

OBESITY LEADS TO SERIOUS HEALTH PROBLEMS

Obese people tend to develop cancer more than lean people. The American Cancer Society has published a study in which they found cancer deaths overall were 33 percent higher for men and 53 percent higher for women whose weight was 40 percent or more above average.[2]

Overweight men have a much higher chance of dying of colon, rectal, and prostate cancer.

Overweight women have higher rates of endometrial, gallbladder, cervical, ovarian, and breast cancer. In breast cancer, obesity is double trouble: Overweight women have an increased risk of getting the disease and a greater likelihood of fatality because fat makes it harder to detect tumors early. A Nurses' Health Study found that women who are forty-four pounds overweight doubled their risk of breast cancer, and a Yale study found that severely obese women were more than three times as likely to be diagnosed late.[3]

High levels of insulin in the bloodstream, a common occurrence among the obese, tends to cause a constant detrimental change in genetic expression, increasing the risk of cancer. In addition, insulin causes too much sodium to be reabsorbed, thereby potentially increasing blood pressure. (There's more on these insulin effects later in this book.)

Both men and women who are overweight often die prematurely, primarily through heart disease, but also through stroke and diabetes—both of which are impacted negatively by excess fat. Obesity puts a person at a much higher risk for developing coronary artery disease, gallbladder disease, kidney disease, liver damage, and other serious health problems—the kind that lead to premature death.

Complications of pregnancy are also more common in overweight individuals. Obese women are less fertile and twice as likely to give birth to babies with spina bifida.

Obesity has been linked to arthritis, gout, and even cataracts.

More General Sickness, Colds, and Flu

Even if you claim not to fear developing a major disease or ailment as a result of obesity, you should know that excess weight greatly impacts a person's immune system. Obesity increases the body's resistance to insulin and its susceptibility to infection. The result is plain and simple: Obese people get sick more often than thin people. If for no other reason, choose to lose the excess fat in your body so you can enjoy more days of good health a year. I promise you will be glad you did!

Overweight people statistically suffer from more colds and infections than lean people. One of the reasons for suppressed immunity in larger people is that the two major organs of the immune system, the thymus and the spleen, are often smaller in the morbidly obese. When the spleen and thymus are too small for the body, the immune system suffers. Immune cells are initially produced in bone marrow and released into the bloodstream. When some of these unspecialized immune cells find their way to the thymus, they mature into specialized T cells. These cells are then programmed to attack substances that are foreign to the body. Other unspecified cells find their way to the spleen, where they develop into macrophages. As the blood filters through the spleen, macrophages literally engulf and digest viruses and bacteria.

Obese people tend to have excess levels of glucose, insulin, adrenocorticotropin ACTH, and corticosterone, and lower levels of growth hormone in their bloodstream. These out-of-whack levels inhibit young unspecified immunity cells from developing into mature macrophages, which again decreases the efficiency of the immune system. Needless to say, sickness and disease are the byproducts of a chronically fatigued immune system.

More Pain

I have yet to see a person who weighs three hundred pounds who does not have joint, ligament, or general body-organ problems. Most complain of ongoing back and knee problems. Obesity—even moderate obesity—puts undue stress on the legs, back, and internal organs. These structural and internal problems compromise a person's mobility and flexibility. In a word, obesity results in *pain*. It limits human motion and the quality of life a person enjoys.

A Serious "Identity" Hit

And finally, obesity can have negative psychological consequences because our society—whether right or not—tends to equate beauty, intelligence, sociability, and even success with thinness. The general prevailing opinion of our society is that those who are obese are undisciplined, unmotivated, and in some way "out of control." It is not surprising that employers tend to hire those who are thin at rates higher than they hire those who are not. The hidden opinion that is rarely expressed seems to be, "If this person can't control his food intake, why should I trust him with my business?"

CONSIDER FAT TO BE ENEMY NUMBER ONE

Fat is an enemy to your health, to your quality of life, and to your success in society.

Note specifically that I said "fat." Not "weight."

Overall body *weight* is determined by muscle, bone, water, and fat. It is excess *fat* that is the culprit associated with health problems. It is the percentage of fat in your body, not the overall weight number you see on the scale, that should become your targeted enemy.

The distinction between fat and weight is critical. Most diet plans on the market today are aimed at overall weight loss, not necessarily fat loss. There's a huge difference. Weight loss can occur with loss of water from the body, loss of muscle mass, and loss of vital-organ tissue! Fat loss must become your goal.

Let's face it. Most weight-loss programs don't work—at least not over the long haul. If you are like many of the clients I see, you've already tried one or more diet plans and the net result was that you may have lost some weight temporarily, but you are likely fatter today than the day you started each of those plans. Yo-yo dieting and periodic crash-dieting programs simply don't work as a life plan.

National surveys estimate that at any given time, from one-quarter to one-half of all adult Americans are on some sort of diet. As a nation we spend more than thirty billion dollars each year on diet aids and remedies, and that number is also rising. The statistics also tell us that 60 percent of those who lose weight regain the pounds they have lost within three to five years, and a high percentage of those people actually gain back more weight.

Permanent fat loss is what this book is all about. Not a temporary fix. Not something you can accomplish in a couple of weeks. Not something that is necessarily the easy way out. But definitely a program that works—works for virtually all people and works for a lifetime!

HOW FAT IS OBESE?

Obesity is, very simply, defined medically as an excess of body fat. Usually, however, obesity is a term that applies to those who are 20 percent over the normal weight for their age, sex, build, and height. Again, that's at least one in three of us and the ranks are growing all the time in spite of the so-called fitness craze that has gripped our nation in recent decades.

The Mayo Clinic in Rochester, Minnesota, also takes into consideration the distribution of weight and whether it places the person at increased risk for certain diseases, and considers whether the person has a medical problem for which a physician recommends weight loss. The conclusion that is nearly always drawn, however, is that those who are more than 20 percent overweight tend to have a distribution of weight that puts excess pressure on the heart and abdominal organs.

And what is the weight that is subject to distribution? The organs of the body and the muscles of the body are fixed in place. It is *fat* that is stashed away in various lumps and cavities of the body. It is *fat* that gives a unique distribution of weight.

Again, it is excess fat that makes us unhealthy, not necessarily excess *weight*. So how much excess fat results in obesity?

For healthy women, fat should not exceed 25 percent of body weight—for men that percentage is 17. (God seemed to design women's bodies to carry a higher percentage of fat tissue to ensure that the body has plenty of fuel for pregnancy and nursing, even if food is scarce. In addition, female fat distribution is designed to help cushion a fetus on impact during pregnancy. That is why the hips and abdominal area enlarge when a woman is pregnant.)

Female reader, if more than 25 percent of your body weight is fat, you are *overfat*.

Male reader, if more than 17 percent of your body weight is fat, you are *overfat*.

Rather than assume at this point that you are *not* overfat because you don't know your body's fat percentage, I suggest you assume that you *are* overfat. And if you aren't, there's a huge likelihood that someone you know and love is.

You should also assume that even if you don't have a fat problem today, you may very well develop one as you grow older.

Get armed with the facts about fat and fat-loss. Get motivated to fight the war against your own excess fat. And get ready for a new way of living that can result in better health, not only in the very near future, but every year for the rest of your life.

HOW THIS PROGRAM DIFFERS FROM ALL OTHERS

This program is not like anything else you have read.

First, it has been proven over a period of more than thirty years of implementation. It isn't something dreamed up, schemed up, or drummed up.

Second, it is based on genuine scientific and medical research. My academic background is in science—biology, chemistry, biochemistry, and psychology. My clinical background is in nutrition and exercise physiology. You may not read all the references in the notes at the end of this book, but you can trust the fact that these are only selected references from thousands I could have chosen and they reflect sound scientific and medical research.

Most of the diet plans that have been published—even the official government position of pushing a high-carbohydrate, low-fat diet—are based on selected pieces of the nutritional puzzle rather than the whole picture of what makes a person healthy. Two of the most important missing pieces of that puzzle involve basal metabolic rate and the two key hormones that govern the way the human body burns calories and stores fat. This program takes into account *all* the pieces of the fat-loss puzzle.

Third, this program reflects a *comprehensive* plan that you can live with the rest of your life.

Most weight-loss plans focus on a particular food group, or a particular supplement, or on one or two quick-fix ideas that seem "catchy." This program deals with what you eat and when, what you drink, what you refuse to eat and drink, how you exercise and when, how often you eat, and which nutritional supplements work best.

One of the things I've discovered, and most of my clients have also discovered, is that good habits tend to build on one another.

There's a synergistic effect. If I work out regularly, I tend to eat right, I work more efficiently, my schedule flows better, and I sleep well. If I eat right, of course, I have more energy for my physical workouts and my business work. If I do all things in sync, it is easier to lose the fat and keep it off.

All of which is to say you will experience the maximum benefit of the fat-loss program outlined in this book when you do all the facets of it simultaneously as a *total program.*

And doesn't that make sense?

Being overfat is something that impacts all facets of your life. Being lean *also* impacts all facets of your life. Getting from overfat to lean requires twelve key changes that encompass all facets of your life.

Are you ready to get started on those changes? The choice to say yes is an important one.

CHOICES AND CONSEQUENCES

As a biochemist and nutritionist, I have a very strong conviction: We live our lives one choice at a time. Every good choice we make helps build a foundation for a good life tomorrow, next year, a decade from now, and perhaps several decades from now.

We each must take responsibility for the choices we make regarding our health. The pursuit of maximum fat loss is a *choice*—a very personal and critically important choice.

I'll never forget the day in tenth grade when it dawned on me that I could look better and feel better than I did. I certainly didn't know what I know today about fat loss, good nutrition, or a healthy way of living, but I did know enough to know that I needed to take personal responsibility for my health and dietary choices.

Years later, in the aftermath of a nearly fatal heart condition, I made more choices about how to regain my health. In the decades that have followed, I have continued to make choices, based on ever-increasing research into nutrition, exercise, and the overall keys to good health. I don't expect my doctor to tell me how to achieve good health. Most physicians are trained in the treatment of disease, only a few are trained in the prevention of disease. Very few people are academically trained to tell people how to achieve the greatest health. Very few understand the body's systems and how they respond to nutritional factors and biochemical influences. I am grateful for every personal discovery I make in this field, and even more importantly, I choose to apply what I know works based on scientific evidence.

Many people know some of the basics of good nutrition and a healthy lifestyle. Far fewer actually put into practice what they know. *Choose* to be a person who will apply the information in this book. *Make a choice* to become personally informed and personally responsible for the best possible health you can achieve.

Knowledge converts to wisdom with repeated application. The truly wise people in this world are those who develop good habits based upon the best possible knowledge.

I hope you are at the point where you will do whatever it takes to lose the excess fat you have stored in your body, because ultimately, maximum fat loss is a personal choice you make. I will give you the basics in this book. You must choose to apply them. I hope you will make that choice today.

And if you really are ready to begin, then the place to begin, as with most things in life, is in the mind.

THE TWELVE VITAL KEYS TO MAXIMUM FAT LOSS

Key #1: Develop a deep desire to do whatever it takes to lose your excess fat.

Key #2: Set realistic goals and motivating rewards.

Key #3: Eat six meals a day, with a calorie total not exceeding ten times your ideal body weight.

Key #4: Eat sufficient high-quality protein at every meal.

Key #5: Eat low-glycemic-index carbohydrates at every meal.

Key #6: Purge your life of the foods and beverages that are bad for you.

Key #7: Drink half your weight in ounces of pure water every day.

Key #8: Take in sufficient fiber every day.

Key #9: Eat essential fatty acids at every meal.

Key #10: Do cardiovascular (aerobic) exercise five times a week for twenty-five minutes in the morning before eating anything.

Key #11: Do strength-building (weight) exercises and flexibility (stretching) exercises three to five times a week.

Key #12: Take supplements daily to help you fight fat and to give your body all the nutrients it needs.

KEY #1:

Develop a deep desire to do whatever it takes to lose your excess fat.

1

FACE UP TO
THOSE FAT CELLS

A high school friend of mine went to both my church and school
and we were in athletics together. We were both strong and in
great shape. Ironically, both of his parents were morbidly obese. I
often wondered how he could be in such good shape when his parents were not.

Twenty years passed between our graduation from high school
and our next meeting. The man I saw twenty years later was not the
teenager I knew. He was as obese as his parents had been, with a belly
just as large as the ones they had when we were boys.

He was not the only one. I was shocked at the number of people
in my graduating class who had become overweight even though
they were thin in high school. Many of those who had been moder-
ately overweight in high school had become morbidly obese!

I can almost hear some of you saying, "It's genetics! He couldn't
help it. Your other friends couldn't help it. It's genetics!"

Here's the reality. Only 20 percent of our body weight is determined by genetics. The remaining 80 percent is determined by our
diet and lifestyle choices.

Parents *teach* their children how and what to eat, not necessarily
by direct teaching methods, but by the example they themselves set.
My friend's youthful levels of testosterone and his high metabolism

born of his athletic activities had kept him thin. But he had learned to eat at his parents' table. As an adult he continued to eat the way he had been taught to eat, and that eating pattern was conducive to massive fat gain.

My friend Zig Ziglar tells the story of a woman who grew up cutting off a narrow slice from the end of her pot roast before she put the roast in the oven. The slice of meat was just tossed away. Her daughter grew up and when she cooked a pot roast, she did the same thing. One day the daughter asked her mother, "Mom, why do we cut off this perfectly good piece of meat at the end of the pot roast before we put the pan in the oven?"

The mother replied, "Well, that's the way Grandma does it."

The daughter asked, "Why does Grandma do that?"

The mother said, "I really have no idea. Let's call her and find out." When they got Grandma on the line this was her explanation: "Oh, I cut off that narrow strip of the pot roast because my roasting pan was too small for the whole piece of meat!"

This family had wasted pounds and pounds of perfectly good beef through the years because of Grandma's undersized roasting pan! Dietary and cooking habits are taught to us as children. That is why it is so important for you to teach your children proper habits.

Do you automatically bread meat before frying it? Do you smother every casserole with cheese? Do you think a person doesn't like what you have cooked if he or she fails to take a second helping? Do you think of the ideal breakfast as bacon and eggs with buttered and jellied white-bread toast? Do you think a meal is incomplete without a piece of pie or cake or a serving of ice cream? Do you drink a large glass of whole milk at every meal?

These are only a few of the many common habits of families that have eaten the same way through the generations . . . and in the process, have eaten their way to obesity.

I've also noticed through the years that obese people tend to have obese cats and dogs as pets. Trust me, there is absolutely no genetic tie-in there. When cats and dogs eat according to the patterns of their obese owners—in quantities that are too large and items that are fattening—they become obese, too.

Now I'm not saying that some people are not predisposed to put on more weight than others. Researchers at Rockefeller University in New York discovered a gene in mice that, if defective, leads to obesity. When activated, this gene apparently produces a hormonelike protein that is secreted by the fat cells into the bloodstream. The mouse gene in which this was found is said to be 85 percent like its human counterpart gene. This discovery may eventually lead to the development of a drug to battle obesity, and it does lend some credence to the theory that some people are more predisposed to put on weight than others.

However—and this is a huge however—the effects of this genetic predisposition can be *counteracted* by behavior. Even if you have this gene in your body, you can choose not to be obese. Remember, as I mentioned earlier, 80 percent of the way genes are expressed is owed to environmental variables! All of us have predispositions to one thing or another; some things are just built into us as human beings. Our behavior, including the acts related to what we put into our mouths and how we choose to exercise, are subject to the human will and to the development of physical habits.

Rather than give in to a genetic predisposition and shrug your shoulders and say, "Well, that's just the way I am," choose to fight this predisposition and say, "This is not the way God originally intended the human body to function and I'm going to make wise choices that give me control over this gene, rather than have this gene control me."

Let me give you a good example related to this.

Many people seem to feel they need something sweet after a meal. I call this the dessert syndrome. There's no genetic predisposition at work in this syndrome. This syndrome is acquired through years of having dessert and of being told that dessert is good after every meal. In many cultures around the world, sweet foods are reserved for rare special occasions, and even then, they tend to be less sweet-tasting that many of the foods Americans gorge themselves on every day.

To break the dessert syndrome, you simply need to say, "I'm going to do something *else* at the conclusion of a meal in place of dessert." Find a new behavior—develop a new after-dinner habit. It may be lingering over a hot cup of green tea without any artificial sweetener (more on this later) and having good conversation time with your spouse or children. It may be taking your big glass of water, flavored with a little fresh lemon juice, out on the deck to enjoy the sunset. It may be moving to the living room for a few minutes of lighting the fireplace and relaxing in front of it, giving yourself the wonderful privilege of ten minutes of downtime or reading.

It may take you several weeks to break the dessert syndrome, but if you diligently attempt to reprogram your own mind regarding this, you will eventually find that you no longer miss sweets. (It is also very important, of course, not to bring desserts home from the grocery store in the first place.)

By the way, an amazing thing happens to our taste buds when we eliminate sugar and the overuse of salt from an eating plan. You'll find that you suddenly discover the real taste of many foods. Years of sugar and salt overexposure dull a person's sense of taste. For those who diligently pursue a fat-loss eating plan, new taste sensations are one of the positive side effects.

I remember hearing one woman wax eloquent about the great taste of farmer's market organic lettuce. I had to suppress a smile as she went on and on about the great taste of the various types of lettuce and greens she had purchased. She had smothered her lettuce salads in so much salad dressing through the years that she had forgotten what lettuce actually tastes like when it is freshly picked and free of chemical washes.

The conclusion to be drawn is this: You do not *need* to be fat. You were not *made* to be fat. You can *decide* that you are going to lose your excess fat and become lean. You can *decide* to make changes in what you eat and how you exercise. You have that ability and that option to *decide*.

YOU CAN CHOOSE TO EMPTY YOUR FAT CELLS

The average human body has between thirty and forty billion fat cells, each of them available to be filled—and crying to be filled. The more fat cells in your body, the easier it is to gain weight.

Now, if we ate like our ancient ancestors, those fat cells would be highly useful to us for storing fat in times when game and edible vegetation were scarce. There are some researchers who believe that our seemingly insatiable love of high-calorie and especially fatty foods may be the remnant of a survival tactic from ancient days when we needed to store fat for future energy.

In our modern society, however, storing energy as fat is no longer necessary for most people. Very few Americans need to go an average of more than three or four hours between meals or snacks. The result? Instead of being a valuable survival mechanism, the body's fat cells become a liability.

A certain number of fat cells are determined by genetic tendency, and others by early eating patterns in a child's life. But let me quickly add that you can't blame your parents entirely for the number of fat cells you have! And furthermore, what you do with those fat cells is up to you.

Through the years I have met a number of people who believe their obesity is related to some kind of glandular malfunction or to a food allergy. Only in very rare cases has that turned out to be true. In some cases, diabetes and hypoglycemia are the root cause of obesity—and in these cases, the more a person controls his blood sugar levels, the greater the weight loss. I still remember taking a physiology course at Florida State University and hearing one of the professors tell us that there was no such thing as glandular obesity. The real causes of obesity in most people are these: emotional tension, boredom, a simple love of food, and basic overeating of the wrong kinds of foods. Poor eating patterns are the number one factor in obesity. Unfortunately, more and more of the wrong kinds of foods are appearing on our supermarket shelves every year.

The fact is, 80 percent of what you look like, no matter how hard you exercise, depends on what you eat. Any type of food that you eat will consistently show up on your body. Trust me on this. Growing up in Florida means that I grew up very conscious about how a person looks in beachwear. There isn't a lot of the body to hide while wearing today's swimsuits so I know—what you eat consistently shows up! I remember telling my friends in college, who were amazed at my low body fat levels and high level of fitness, "You can work out all you want, but until you control your diet, you will never lower your body-fat level."

I often say to people that it doesn't matter nearly so much what they eat between Christmas and New Year's as what they eat from New Year's to Christmas. It is our eating *pattern* that creates body size and the distribution of fat in the body.

Not only do we want a free lunch, but we want it served immediately upon order. And not only do we want a fast free lunch, but we want it to have no calories. Life simply doesn't work that way.

I'm amazed at people who want to watch 4.4 hours of television a day, eat anything in sight, lounge around until noon on Saturdays and then go to a movie and drink a giant sugared soda and eat a massive tub of buttered popcorn . . . and who then wonder why they are overweight. So many people are looking for a magic pill that will make fat go away without any effort whatsoever on their part. Again, life doesn't work that way.

We seem to have lost the concept that self-restraint and self-discipline are virtues. Certainly I'm not calling for rigid self-denial or strict asceticism, but rather a return to the words *moderation* and *personal responsibility*. Maybe the terms *gluttony, self-indulgence,* and *sloth* need to be reintroduced to our vocabulary, to replace euphemisms like "big eaters" and "people with hearty appetites."

REFUSE TO LIVE IN DENIAL

Obesity and good health cannot coexist. To believe anything else is to live in denial. I don't care how you attempt to justify your excess fat to me, I won't buy your argument. I know too much about fat and what it does to the human body.

I have had people say to me, "Well, I'm not obese. I'm only about forty pounds overweight." Friend, that's obese.

There are others who say, "Well, I may have excess fat but I'm in good health. I never get sick." Perhaps you don't catch every virus that comes to your city but you are *not* well at a cellular or tissue level. You are very likely experiencing some type of cardiovascular or joint problems, even if you haven't had any medical tests or symptoms to prove it.

Several years ago as I stood in line at an airline counter, I witnessed a very disturbing scene. Several people were in line ahead of me and each member of the group was purchasing a ticket for a particular flight. It was evident that one of the women was obese and would simply not fit into a standard coach seat. The ticket agent quietly suggested that the woman might be more comfortable if she purchased two seats. The woman became very angry at this suggestion and loudly told the agent that she did not appreciate the implication that she was too large and she did not like being treated rudely in front of her friends. The more the ticket agent tried to calm her down and reason with her, the more angry the woman became. After several minutes of arguing and discussing the situation with one of the airline managers, the woman was given the necessary extra seat at no additional charge.

Talk about denial.

Many people who are obese don't *believe* they are obese, and they are in even greater denial about their need to do anything about it.

I have a friend who probably weighs between four-and five hundred pounds—he won't tell me exactly how much he weighs. I said to him not too long ago, "You know, you might want to consider Bariatric surgery. You have a real problem with obesity."

"No, no," he countered. "I can handle it."

The fact is he isn't handling it. He has shoulder problems, back problems, ankle problems, and knee problems. He can hardly do any physical exertion whatsoever without huffing and puffing. If I strapped a three-hundred-pound weight to my body, I'd have the same problems he's having—all kinds of joint problems, back problems, and breathing problems.

Our bodies are simply not designed to carry around massively excessive amounts of fat. We were created to be lean.

If you are obese, face up to the fact that you are obese.

Admit that if you don't do something about your obesity, you are going to reap consequences that are far from pleasant. You may already be reaping some of them, but you most assuredly are going to reap even more negative consequences in the future.

Admit to yourself: "I am obese and I am ruining my own health."

But don't stop there. Add an important line: "I am going to make a decision to turn this around and to refuse to live out the myth I've bought into."

REFUSE TO LIVE OUT A FAT MYTH

We've all heard the phrase "a big, fat lie." Well, for many people a lie is at the root of their excessive fat. They have bought into a widespread myth that some people are just destined to be fat.

"I'm Fat Because I'm a Woman."

That's a myth. Don't blame your sex for your fat.

It is true that women store fat in different places than men. Women have more fat-deposit areas on their buttocks and in the upper legs. Men carry more fat deep within their abdominal cavity; women carry fat in the abdomen just below the surface of the skin.

Gender hormones are responsible for these fat-storage areas, and there's nothing you can do about that fact. Women after menopause, however, begin to carry their fat in ways that are more like a man.

It is also true that women can have about 8 percent more body fat than men and still be healthy. That extra percentage is *not* an excuse, however, for being fat. Obesity is never an automatic destiny for any woman.

"I'm Fat Because I Have a Slow Metabolism."

Part of your *battle* against fat has to do with metabolism. It is not an automatic destiny, however, that you have a slow metabolism and can do nothing to change it. That's a myth.

Recognize that you have been given a unique body and a unique glandular system and metabolism. We have all seen illustrations of what the body's organs are supposed to look like. Each of us has unique variations on that general theme. Only rarely is the size and shape of a heart that comes from an autopsied body the same size and shape of hearts in textbooks.

Also consider the fact that, theoretically, a person is supposed to have twenty-one feet of small intestine. What about the person who has twenty-three feet? That person is able to absorb 10 percent more of each meal he eats. And the person with only nineteen feet of intestine? That person likely can eat more because his body is rather inefficient (in comparison to the norm) at extracting nutrients from the food he eats.

The body you have been given is your *starting* point. It need not be your *ending* point. If you have a slow metabolism, you can rev it up! If you have inherited a propensity toward more fat cells, you can refuse to fill them with fat. If you have inherited a large bone structure, good for you! You can carry more muscle on those bones and still be lean.

Refuse to blame your obesity on your own anatomy or physiology. My own family is of European descent My maternal grandmother's family, the Kosmeiers, are large people. My mother often tells me, "You are like my side of the family." I guess she means that if I allowed myself I could easily become overweight. No, thank you.

"I Just Can't Seem to Diet."

Refuse to give in to the lie that you are a failure at dieting and that losing fat is an impossibility.

Choose to learn from your past experiences. If you haven't lost the weight you desired to lose on past fat-loss plans, or if you haven't been able to sustain a weight loss in the past, make adjustments. Don't think you can follow the same nutrition, exercise, and supplementation program you did in the past and get different results. If you want different results, you have to take a different approach!

I recall hearing Venus Williams comment on her win in the finals of the U.S. Open Women's tennis tournament in 2000. She had been down 1-4 in the first set and things were not going her way. She commented, "I made a couple of adjustments in my game and things started going my way." Those adjustments were major! She won the next six games in a row, not only winning the set but setting herself up to win the second set and the match. (By the way, I am a big Williams sisters fan. I worked with both Venus and Serena as a nutritionist several years ago when they were training at Greenleaf, Florida.)

You may not need to change *everything* about the way you seek to lose fat. Three or four adjustments may be the key to turning things around.

Choose to believe the *truth* about your obesity. It isn't a matter of your sex, your physiology, or your inability. It's a matter of *choices*—decisions—that have developed into *habits* in your life. The more you continue to make bad choices, the more you reinforce bad habits.

DECIDE TO GET OUT OF YOUR FAT RUT

Most people do not deliberately choose the ruts they live in. They adopt a certain set of habits fairly early in life, or early in their careers, and they continue to plow that rut. Making a change in the way you eat and exercise means plowing a new furrow in your life— it means making an intentional choice about how you are going to live from this point onward.

Some habits we get from our parents, some from our close friends, some from our coworkers, and some we seem to invent on our own. Very often, these habits follow the course of least resistance. We do what feels easy or quick. We like patterns of behavior that require as little effort and as little thought as possible. At the core of all obesity is not simply a set of bad exercise and eating habits, but a failure to think long and hard and to make an active decision about exercise and eating. It always amazes my wife Sharon when she goes to dinner with a friend and the friend tries to get her to eat something unhealthy "because Ted's not here." When she turns down the junk food they often act surprised. I guess folks forget that my wife and I both practice what we preach and that she has written a best-selling natural-foods cookbook.

Hopefully no one chooses to be obese (except for Sumo wrestlers). But we do choose the activities and behaviors that make us obese.

Choose to make a new choice!

Virtually all people in our culture have a choice of what they are going to eat, when they are going to eat, how much they are going to eat, and how much or whether they are going to exercise. We have a great deal of freedom of choice in our nation about how much fat we are going to carry around on our bodies.

We have no freedom of choice when it comes to the consequences associated with retention of excess fat in our bodies. Those consequences are set; we may not experience them immediately, but we will experience them eventually if we fail to remove the excess fat.

If you step off the roof of a ten-story building, stating that you do not believe in the law of gravity and that you refuse to accept the consequences associated with the law of gravity, you are going to plummet to your death in spite of what you believe or choose to accept. The laws of nature are fixed, including the laws of nature regarding your health.

If you neglect your physical health and allow yourself to become and remain morbidly obese, you *will* suffer the consequences of ill health.

Your first step, then, toward a lasting fat-loss program is to decide that *you* are going to change the way you have been living *for the better*. Let's face it, if you are twenty-to thirty-or even forty pounds over fat and you continue to practice the bad habits that made you this way, you are going to continue to get the same results.

Note those two areas that are italicized in the preceding paragraph: *You*, and only you, have the power to make a change in your life. You, and only you, can motivate yourself to make that change a lasting change that is *for the better*. If you are intent on losing fat to please anybody other than yourself, your motivation is going to rise and fall on that person's approval of you, love for you, or acceptance of you. Lose fat because you decide that this is the right thing to do for you.

TURN YOUR DECISION INTO A HEART'S DESIRE

Deep down inside, you need to come up with a driving reason for why you want to make this decision to lose fat. That's the key to turning a decision into a desire. A desire is more deeply rooted in a person's life. A desire has an emotional component attached to it. A desire compels changes in attitude and behavior. When losing fat becomes your heart's desire, you will start to do something about your obesity. I remember when I made this choice as a fifteen-year-old sophomore in high school. I had had enough of being fat. I chose to start working out, and to change the way I ate. *The change has to begin with you!*

Let me offer you seven good reasons that can turn a decision into a desire:

Reason #1

You want to be in better health, not only today and tomorrow but in the future. The end result is that you want to live longer and enjoy a better quality of life. The sub-reasons may be that you can overcome some of the pain and discomfort you presently feel. When you are sick of being sick . . . you *will* act!

Reason #2

You want to look better. The end result is likely to be greater sociability and success. The sub-reasons for this may also be many—from feeling better in your clothes to putting yourself into a better position for a raise or new job. When you don't like what you see in your own mirror and when your self-identity is at stake . . . you *will* act.

Reason #3

You want to have more energy. Those who carry around no extra fat and who are eating the right foods to sustain a fat-free life tend to have far more energy. When you become tired of being tired all the time . . . you *will* act.

Reason #4

When you become truly convinced that God both desires the best for you and wants you to be lean . . . you *will* act.

Reason #5

You want to prevent as many health problems as possible so you can enjoy your later years to their fullest. Good health habits started as a young person, or even as a middle-aged person, pay off huge dividends as a person reaches retirement years. The sub-reasons for this may be many: so you can see your grandchildren grow up, so you can go places you long to visit in your retirement, so you can avoid living in a nursing home. When you have a renewed zest for living life to the fullest and to a ripe old age . . . you *will* act.

Last month I had an ultrasound scan of my carotid artery. I wanted to see if I am as healthy internally as I am externally. This type of scan shows if you have any plaque build-up in your artery. This is a good indication of overall cardiovascular health. I am happy to announce that when the results came back they revealed that I have zero—that's right *zero*—plaquing in my artery. In other words, my cardio-vascular system is in great shape. I highly recommend this scan to everyone.

Reason #6

You want to improve your social life. People tend to gravitate toward those who have vitality—a real enthusiasm for life, deep joy, and a lean body weight. When you want to feel closer to people, or perhaps to just one person . . . you *will* act.

Reason #7

You have a deep inner conviction that this is the right thing to do *now* and not later. Most people who are overweight know deep down inside that they should do something about their excess fat and that today is the best day to start a fat-loss program. When you have a real urgency that you need to get lean *now* . . . you *will* act.

Do you know what you want? I learned through an informal survey in my office that 97 percent of those who made New Year's resolutions didn't keep them because they hadn't made resolutions that truly reflected what they wanted in their lives. The fact is, we do what we desire to do. If you aren't doing certain things, the reason is simple: You don't truly *desire* to do them.

Don't merely make a decision. Develop a desire.

As part of developing a desire, you may need to trade in some of your old attitudes for new ones. . .

2

IF YOUR OLD ATTITUDES AND IDEAS HAVEN'T WORKED . . . TRADE THEM IN!

I remember an over-fat friend of mine in college who once told me, "I'll eat right and start exercising after I graduate and have more time." As you may have guessed, after graduation he never changed and is obese today.

A fat-loss program is about change. And change is about being open and about releasing old ideas that really aren't working for you.

If your old ideas about eating have led you to become obese . . . you need some new ideas about eating.

If your old ideas about exercising have led you to become sedentary and overweight . . . you need some new ideas about exercise.

If your antiquated ideas about drinking enough water have led you to be sick all the time and to retain even more water weight . . . you need some new ideas about how much water you should drink in a day.

If your ideas about supplementation are limited to a super-cheap daily multiple vitamin tablet . . . you need some new ideas about adequate supplementation and purchasing top-quality vitamins, minerals, and other nutrients.

If your ideas have led to a you that you don't like to see in the mirror . . . it's time to get some new ideas for creating the you that you desire to be!

The link between a powerful body and a powerful mind has been recognized for ages. The ancient Greeks were convinced that a person could only unlock his full potential when the intellect and the body reached a harmonious balance. That was the philosophy behind the creation of the Greek gymnasium—a place to exercise both body and mind. The Romans had a phrase they used in their admiration of the Greeks: *Mens sana in corpore sano*—which means "a sound mind in a sound body."

The way you look definitely impacts the self-image you have of yourself. And conversely, the way you think about yourself, and about your own body and health, impacts what you do to improve your physique and health.

Your attitude is the unseen factor in achieving and maintaining maximum fat loss. Set your attitude meter on the highest positive level!

DUMP ALL YOUR OLD EXCUSES

People use countless excuses to remain fat. Here are some of the many I've heard:

- When I'm fat I don't have to deal with advances from the opposite sex. (This is probably true!)
- My spouse will become jealous if I lose weight and become more attractive to other people. (Trust me, your spouse will be happy.)
- People will think I'm ill or have AIDS if I lose too much weight. (Just tell them you finally found a fat-loss program that works.)
- If I lose weight I'll have more wrinkles. (Maybe a few.)
- I'm too old to care about how I look. (Bad attitude!)

- My fat is inherited. (Yeah, right.)

- I'm fat primarily because I've had babies. (Hormonal changes can be corrected.)

- Eating is my greatest pleasure—take away food and I won't have much joy in life. (You need to get a life.)

- My life is too stressful right now to diet—I can't add one more concern to my life, much less my body fat. (If you don't make fat-loss a concern, you may not have a life at all!)

- My doctor has said I have too many fat cells and too slow a metabolism; I must be incurably fat. (Get another doctor.)

- It will take forever to lose all the weight I should, and I just can't see myself maintaining a program that long. (You have the rest of your life.)

- I've been on lots of diets and I always seem to gain the weight back. (Bad choice of programs.)

- I don't like to cook and plan menus, and that's what dieting is all about. (Get my wife's cookbook.)

- My work forces me to eat out a lot and I can't imagine losing weight when eating in restaurants all the time. (Make better menu choices.)

- My friends would never put up with a special diet. (Find new friends who care about your health.)

- Food means love, comfort, and security to me—take away food and I don't know where I'd turn for pleasure and feelings of safety. (How about your loved ones?)

- I'm not good at making changes. (Well, *get* good!)

Just how many excuses are there for not beginning a fat-loss program? I'm not sure any of us has the time or energy to count that high! I've heard more excuses than I care to recall, but nearly all of them end with one of these phrases:

"I'll start next Monday."

"I'm making it my New Year's resolution."

"I'll do it after my vacation."

Procrastination, procrastination, procrastination.

There always seems to be something that keeps us from starting that fat-loss program *today*.

Many people wait for things to be "perfect" in their lives before they take a positive step toward fat loss. You guessed it—perfection never arrives. Don't wait until New Year's Day. Don't wait for Monday. Don't wait for the start of a new month. Don't wait for the full moon to rise, the tide to turn, or the end of summer vacation. Start today!

SEE YOURSELF IN A NEW LIGHT

The day has come for you to see yourself as *extraordinary*, not just ordinary. The average person in our society has a weight problem and is doing nothing about it. Choose not to be average or ordinary for another day.

Choose to be uniquely and distinctively all that you can be.

Most people need to make five serious attitude adjustments in order to see themselves as extraordinary and capable of getting lean and staying lean.

Attitude Adjustment #1: I do have enough self-discipline.

So many people groan, "I just don't have the self-discipline I need to lose weight."

Yes, they do. And so do you.

We all have great self-discipline . . . in pursuing our existing patterns and habits. Through years of repeated "doing," we have disciplined ourselves to reach for certain things, go to certain restaurants, order certain dishes, sit in certain easy chairs, and engage in other patterns of behavior that we rarely dream of altering.

Discipline does not only pertain to good patterns of behavior. Discipline means strictly following a code of behavior that you have established for yourself. It can be a good code of behavior or a bad one—that choice is up to you.

I know a man who has disciplined himself very highly to have a dish of ice cream at eight o'clock every evening. I know a woman who has disciplined herself to *call* a person to walk her dog every morning at seven o'clock. (She wouldn't think of walking the dog herself because her hair hasn't been curled at that hour.)

Bad habits can become just as natural and comfortable to your brain as good ones. And once a pattern of behavior is accepted, adopted, and repeated often enough, it becomes *discipline.*

The key to losing fat and maintaining fat loss is to change the habits of daily behavior and to work at changing those habits until they become a new discipline.

Many habits need to be changed, but they can be difficult to change. I won't argue that point with you. However, you must admit that it is exciting to finally adopt a new way of exercising and eating that actually works.

My point is not that life-pattern changes are easy. My point is that the establishment of new habits is doable, and you have the ability and self-discipline to make changes in the way you eat, exercise, and think about eating and exercise.

Through the years I've seen people with doctorate degrees, leaders in business, and very successful people in other fields fail at fat loss. Lack of discipline? Hardly. They had to have a great deal of discipline to achieve the things they have. These people were just disciplined in the wrong behaviors when it came to fat loss!

The key to fat loss lies partly in having the right information—in knowing what to do and in knowing the right combination of behaviors, both to start and maintain a fat-loss program. Knowing what to do and doing what you know are two entirely different things. That's what this book is all about. I know you have the self-discipline. I'm here to give you the information you need to develop new habits that will become your new discipline.

I believe from the bottom of my heart that you have the ability to carry out this plan and to stick with it.

You need to believe it, too.

Attitude Adjustment #2: It's okay to do this solely for myself.

No, you aren't being self-centered, self-absorbed, or egocentric by desiring to lose fat. You are being smart. And you are making a choice to maximize your own potential. There's nothing selfish about wanting to be healthy and look your best.

Several months ago I attended the funeral of a friend who had been fifty pounds overweight. He had always been thinking about helping others. Sadly, he died at the age of fifty-one from a massive heart attack. It's not selfish to want to be healthy so that you can live a long and productive life.

A short time after that funeral, I received word that another overweight friend of my family in Germany had died at the age of forty-one. Again, she was a person who had always thought about others. She wasn't serious about her weight problem. In the end, she hadn't really thought about how devastating her *death* would be to those she claimed to care about most.

You also need to be realistic about the prevailing media messages that manipulate you in subliminal ways to get lean.

Many young women who work as models and television actresses have very short careers. Why don't they survive on camera into their twenties and thirties? The plain fact is that some die. Most, however, don't die—they just become too sick to be beautiful. Those who are anorexic or bulimic become sickly looking over time, even though they may not perceive themselves this way when they look in a mirror. In addition, they have less and less energy and therefore less and less vitality to their "look." Part of the misperception anorexics and bulimics have about themselves can also lead to severe depression, which inhibits their ability to work.

One night not too long ago I saw a television talk show that dealt with "Hollywood's Weight-Loss Plan." The discussion dealt with the ABCs of celebrity weight loss: anorexia, bulimia, caffeine, cigarettes, and cocaine. Without a doubt, those who consume great amounts of caffeine or who smoke, lowering the oxygen level to their skin, destroy their skin tone and become "old" looking way before their time. When it comes to cocaine use, the death statistics start to pile up, along with serious health problems that destroy one's beauty or appearance of fitness.

How many times have you heard of a Hollywood star in rehab for drugs or alcohol? This is a major problem all across the country, and most of it is due to the unrealistic message sent by tall, paper-thin models who have undergone extensive plastic surgery. Be realistic. Not everyone is going to look this way even with plastic surgery. What we all need to focus on is being the best and the healthiest we can be. And *that* is what this book is all about.

Many people, by choosing to undereat, eat-and-purge, or use caffeine, cigarettes, or cocaine as weight-control drugs, are hoping to give themselves a beauty edge. In reality, over time they are destroying the natural beauty they have at the outset of their youth.

Not only do you need to tune out the subliminal message that "extreme thinness" is the look to achieve, but you also need to tune out the message that the way you achieve an overly thin look is through mishandling food or other substances.

At the same time, a "before and after" photo of yourself can be motivating and help you in attitude adjustment. Have a friend take two photos of you—pretty much like full-body police mug shots—one face on and one side view. Stand relatively relaxed with your arms at your sides and wear a swimsuit or shorts and a top that you can tuck into your shorts. Put those photos where you can see them periodically—perhaps by your side of the bed, on your refrigerator door, or in your home gym. Honestly evaluate your own body. It's *you*. You are the one who can make the changes. You are the one responsible. What do you want to change about yourself, for yourself?

Refuse to play a comparison game. There are those who become very smug about what they are doing when it comes to exercise and nutritious eating. It's easy to say to yourself, "Well, I'm doing better than 90 percent of the people on the planet." Yes, but are you doing *all* that you personally can do to achieve maximum fat loss and, in the process, gain maximum health and energy? Do your best, regardless of what others around you may be doing.

More likely is the scenario in which you compare yourself to others and find yourself coming up short. You aren't making as much progress as the next person, you aren't walking as fast, lifting as much weight, losing fat as quickly, or looking as good. Get your eyes off others and onto your own mirror. Are *you* making progress? That's the real question to ask yourself. If you aren't, is there something you need to adjust to make more progress?

Over the years, in countless fitness facilities, I have learned the importance of working on my own goals. There will always be someone who is in better shape or who responds better to exercise. Instead of being upset or jealous about these people, just realize that there may be another area of their life where they may not have had as much "success" as you have. So please stop the comparisons. Unless they are used to positively motivate you they really are counter-productive.

Let me give you an example of how I use comparisons to be motivated. My workout partner is named Van Green. Van is a former NFL defensive back. He and I have been friends for over ten years and workout partners for over four. He is an absolute inspiration to me. He is 6'3", 218 pounds, has 6 percent body fat and can do 27 pull-ups in one set. He still runs like the wind and really pushes me in our workouts. In addition, he is a super-positive ordained minister of the gospel and we constantly encourage one another. I realize that no matter how hard I work out I will never be the athlete Van is. However, I don't allow that comparison to discourage me. I use it to motivate me.

If you are going to choose a workout partner it is better to choose one you don't have to beg to work out. Choose someone who shows up on time and who eats the same types of foods you choose. This makes the workout much more focused and allows you to concentrate on your fitness goals rather than be sidetracked by an unmotivated partner who doesn't want to work out.

During my years of training I have had three workout partners who motivated me: Gene Dawes in 1974, Steve Sanzone in 1976, and Van Green for the last four years. The reason I am telling you this is that for all of the years in between, I worked out primarily by myself. That is why it is so important to be self-motivated. If you always need someone to get you up during a workout, what happens when that person does not show up? Learn to motivate yourself. If you do not know how to work out order my exercise videos from my office (1-800-726-1834). That way I can be your partner, and I'll always show up.

In summary, be glad about your own successes and don't compare them to others'. Rather than think, *Wow, I've only lost fifteen pounds after three months,* choose to think, *Wow! I now weigh fifteen pounds less than I did just ninety days ago! I'm on my way!* In doing so you will have a much better attitude about your life-long health journey.

Attitude Adjustment #3: I can choose to see myself as a winner with a positive outlook.

Take a long hard look at your own attitudes. Do you really have a positive attitude toward losing fat? Do you have a positive attitude about your chances of succeeding at a fat-loss program? Do you have a positive attitude in general?

Until you get your attitude in line, you aren't likely to put on your walking shoes, take control of your eating, or do the other things necessary to achieve maximum fat loss.

Once you have made the consistent choice to look at fat loss in a positive way, take a look at others around you. Your attitude is going to be greatly influenced by those with whom you eat and exercise. How many times have you been out with friends and because they ate too much or weren't concerned about their health you followed in their footsteps?

Another very potent thing you can do to turn off the negative stress in your body is to tune out the negativity and cynicism you are likely to find at just about every turn in our society. TV and newspapers and many magazines are filled with cynicism and news that is mostly negative and really unnecessary.

I am never surprised when people tell me that they lack confidence in their ability to lose fat or that they don't know if they can dare to dream of becoming lean and healthy. Most people are so steeped in negative thinking and cynicism that they don't think positively about *anything* in their lives. I have never actually calculated this in a scientific way, but I believe that most of the obese people I meet are individuals who have set very few goals for themselves in their finances, in their careers, or in any other area of their lives. On the other hand, the people I know who have set and reached and are maintaining fat-loss goals are people who tend to have lots of other goals—from family goals to spiritual-growth goals to financial investment goals.

Cynicism and negativity, time after time, lead to failure. Optimism and confidence lead to success. It's as simple as that. You can see the pattern in person after person if you truly study their lives and get to know their innermost attitudes.

Cynicism is a dangerous mental outlook for any individual. It robs a person of self-motivation and a positive self-image. The cynical person says, "Why try?" "What's the use?" "There's always going to be something to trip me up or someone to beat me at the game." Cynics cry, "It's not worth the effort. Nothing really works as advertised. Physical goals related to weight, leanness, fitness, and health are futile."

I wholeheartedly disagree.

I choose to be *positive* about my life—all aspects of it.

I challenge you to be positive about who God created you to be and about your ability to maximize every area of your life in the pursuit of all your potential!

Turn off the cynics. Turn off the negativity.

I once read an article in which Arnold Schwarzenegger insisted that the positive energy, discipline, determination, and strength he developed through bodybuilding were the keys to his success in virtually every other area of his life—from his rise to the top of the motion-picture industry to his prosperity as a real-estate tycoon to his success as a husband and father.

That's the way I hope you will feel when you make a firm commitment to pursuing and then maintaining a fat-loss program. Turning away from excess fat and ill health and toward a lean, healthy body is a major moment.

There is a great deal you can do personally to address the issue of negative-stress reduction. Faith, if used properly, can be a tremendous negative-stress reducer. In my life an unwavering faith in God gives me tremendous peace of mind. And I've discovered that when my mind and heart are at peace, the stress in my physical body is released. I heartily recommend that a person have a quiet time. Choose to read inspirational books such as Zig Ziglar's and uplifting magazine articles. (I like reading the Bible, especially the book of Proverbs. King Solomon, who compiled the proverbs, is not only credited with being one of the wisest men in the history of the world, but also one of the wealthiest.) Interestingly enough, wisdom provides benefits to every area of our life, including health and finances.

It's far better to eat alone than to eat with a group of people who are down about everything and who have a negative, cynical attitude toward all things that might be associated with success. Negative people tend to be negative about virtually everything, and it won't be long until you'll hear negative comments from them about your fat loss and your new, leaner appearance. "Dear, you are looking so pale these days." "Are you sick?" "You're losing weight much too fast." "Don't be a party spoiler—here, try this dessert." "You don't want to get *too* thin." Yes, it's better to eat alone than to eat with those who try to force their negativity on your fat-loss goals! Ideally, you will find positive friends with whom you can share your meals.

Choose to work out at a gym that is filled with a spirit of optimism, encouragement, and camaraderie. I was fifteen years old, I started working out in just such a gym. Now that I'm forty-five years old I still look back with fond memories on those early gym days. We had fun working out together. Hang out with people who are positive about their own successes and who are quick to encourage your success. It makes a huge difference.

In order to receive positive energy from others, you must give positive energy. Be quick to compliment others. Be quick to encourage those you know who are on a fat-loss program. Write a little note. Make a phone call to say, "Hey, I support what you're doing and I think it's great." If you see a person at the gym on a regular basis and notice that they are making good progress, let them know the next time the two of you are at the water fountain: "Looks like you're making some excellent progress—I admire your hard work." You'll make their day! During my workout today with Van I told him how great his arms look. He did an extra twelve reps. It is amazing what positive words from a friend can do.

Give some positive feedback, too, to your family members who encourage, rather than criticize, your fat-loss efforts. A little note can let your family members know you are grateful that they aren't nagging you, but rather are supportive of you: "I really appreciate your support. It helps me to stay motivated to become all I can be."

What you say to others will not only be encouraging to them, but your own two ears will hear those encouraging words. In speaking positive words to others, you are also taking in a positive message for your own spirit.

Those who you encourage and who encourage you become your support group. A support group can be as small as two people! Your chances of success in any fat-loss program are going to be enhanced if there's at least one other person who will join you in pursuing a healthful eating plan and an exercise program. Even if you can only find a morning walking partner, you'll find it easier to stay with your fat-loss program.

Attitude is extremely important for achieving and then maintaining maximum fat loss. You can lose pounds. But believe me, when you have a positive, "charged-up" attitude toward fat loss, your meal times are going to be more pleasant, your exercise sessions are going to be more invigorating and enjoyable, and your overall success rate is going to be much higher, much faster.

Attitude Adjustment #4: I can accomplish a long-term goal.

First, be reasonable about what you expect to achieve, and by when. A woman once came into my office very eager to start a fat-loss program. She knew exactly how much she wanted to weigh and what size dress she wanted to wear. I asked her, "What percentage of body fat do you expect to have?" (We'll talk more about how to determine this percentage later.)

She stared at me blankly. I knew we were at ground zero and had a long way to go.

Then I asked, "And by when do you hope to achieve your ideal health?" She said, "Oh, in three months. That's when my daughter is getting married."

Her expectations were unreasonable on all counts. I explained to her that even with the most extreme protocol, the greatest amount of effort, and virtual starvation between now and that date, she was not going to achieve her goal. Her face registered disbelief, then dismay, then depression—all in a few seconds. (By the way, she wanted to lose one hundred pounds in three months.)

I quickly moved to encourage her. "What we can do," I said, "is set a more reasonable goal and develop a plan for getting there. What I require of you is not only that you agree to follow the plan, but that you choose to be realistic in your expectations and choose to be happy with the results you achieve in ninety days. If you are happy with the progress you have made at the end of ninety days, the glow of your attitude will more than make up for your dress size."

She agreed and we began to work together.

Set a reasonable goal for yourself as well as a reasonable time frame for achieving your goal.

When I was in my twenties I took my new bride Sharon to the fish camp where I had been raised as a child. Although Sharon had grown up in Florida, she had not grown up near a lake or canal so she had never been around many reptiles. Due to erosion over the years, a lot of roots had surfaced near the trees next to the lake. As my wife was walking near the edge of the water, she stepped on one of those roots only to have it move under her feet. She had inadvertently stepped on a large water moccasin!

The snake immediately took aim. Sharon leaped straight up in the air and began to move her legs like an egg beater even before her feet hit the ground. (She reminded me of Fred Flintstone, the cartoon character, jumping up in the air and getting ready to run!) She ran away from that snake faster than I've ever seen her move, before or since!

Just as obesity doesn't strike you like a snake, neither can you run away from it like you can run from a snake.

There are no quick cures. You are going to have to

- learn how to control your food and fluid intake

- learn how to control your supplemental (vitamins, minerals, and essential fats intake,

- learn how to fold proper exercise into the mix of your daily schedule, and

- learn how to motivate yourself to keep working on your fat-loss goals over time.

A change in your eating patterns and your exercise work together. Changing just your eating, or just your exercise, isn't going to do much for fat loss. Yet another reason why a *comprehensive* plan is necessary!

Attitude Adjustment #5: I do have the courage to overcome my fears about losing weight.

Ask yourself: Am I afraid of positive change? Is there a particular fear that has kept me paralyzed behind my fat? Am I afraid someone may reject me if I change? Am I afraid of missing out on fun times with my friends? Am I afraid of having less energy?

This last fear is one I hear fairly often. Most people have dieted incorrectly in the past and have suffered from hunger pangs and a loss of energy. The fat-loss program outlined in this book, however, is one that is going to increase your energy levels. Let me encourage you to tackle that fear head-on!

IT IS IMPORTANT TO IDENTIFY AND WRITE DOWN POSITIVE ATTITUDES

In addition to the five new attitudes I've suggested to you in this chapter, I recommend that you come up with some positive thoughts of your own. Write them down and then post them where you can see them periodically. They may be such thoughts as

- I'm working for progress, not perfection.
- I'm always in control of my food intake.
- My body is my most valuable possession.
- I always eat to look and feel my best!
- I can do all things through Christ who strengthens me.

The more you fuel your mind with a can-do spirit, the more you can do and will want to do! Speak in positive, affirmative, first-person terms to yourself. Those statements are the most effective!

A set of positive attitudes about yourself and about a fat-loss program is the best possible set-up you can have for the hard cold reality that comes next.

3

JUST *HOW* FAT ARE YOU?— COMPARING WHAT IS WITH WHAT SHOULD BE

Obesity is not subtle. Fat tends to be right out there where you and everybody else can see it. The consequences of obesity can be violent. The fat that builds up over time, however, can seem to be subtle.

One day when my family and I were out on the dock next to the lake where we live, a twelve-foot alligator swam by. Now, it's not a good thing when an alligator swims that close to a dock. It means the alligator has lost all fear of human beings and would just as soon have a child or a family pet for a meal. We called the game wardens, but in spite of a very diligent search and the setting of various traps, neither they nor we could find that 'gator.

Two years later, I was having a conversation with one of our neighbors and the subject of that alligator came up. I asked my neighbor, "Do you know what ever happened to that big 'gator we saw a couple of years ago?"

He said, "Ted, I didn't want to tell anybody for fear of getting in trouble, but that alligator kept coming around the docks. I saw it several times. One time it came up on the beach and settled down to sun itself just a few yards from where some of our grandchildren were playing. I went inside and got my shotgun and killed that alligator. Then I called a friend and he and I hauled it off."

I was grateful.

Now I realize that some of you may be thinking that he shouldn't have killed the alligator. I'd like to remind you that I'm not talking about a manatee or a bald eagle or an endangered species here. I'm talking about a reptile that regularly attacks adults, children, and pets in the state of Florida. If you have never heard that fact before, it's probably because the Florida Department of Tourism doesn't consider it one of Florida's top selling points.

Alligators have a way of lying in wait for their next meal. They can loiter under docks or lie nearly completely submersed in the shallow waters next to a lake's edge and wait there for a long time until an unsuspecting meal comes their way. An alligator attack can be subtle, but vicious nonetheless.

The same goes for the "attacks" that arise from too much fat in the bloodstream. We call them angina attacks or heart attacks if they occur in the coronary vessels; we call them strokes if they occur in the brain. The fat gain leading up to the attack may be subtle, but the attack itself can be vicious and deadly.

Don't wait for that attack moment to come. Get rid of the 'gator of obesity before it attacks you in a deadly or debilitating away.

TAKE INVENTORY OF YOUR OWN BODY

Many weight-management plans begin with the advice: "See your doctor before starting any serious weight-loss plan." The main reason for seeing a doctor is not so the doctor can approve or even applaud your intention of losing weight. The main reason for seeing a physician, as far as I am concerned, is so you can get a set of baseline numbers and measurements that will serve both to motivate you and give you a means of evaluating your progress.

I do *not* recommend that you ask your physician to order tests to determine your fat percentage. An underwater fat-displacement test can be very expensive. You can measure the percentage of fat in your body in the privacy of your own home using a simple device called a *fat caliper.* Owning such a device also allows you to keep better track of your progress through the weeks and months of your fat-loss program. (You can order a fat caliper through our office if you can't find one. Give me a call at 1-800-726-1834.)

Let me make a little aside about what you can expect from your physician: Do not expect your physician to be a weight-loss expert.

I often hear my clients say, "Why hasn't my physician ever told me any of this?" The reason is most physicians are not trained in nutrition or preventive health care. Modern mainstream medicine is pathology oriented—it is primarily concerned with crisis intervention and the resolution of problems "after something has gone wrong" or has "broken." Our physicians, for the most part, are experts in the arenas of pills and scalpels. They are trained to prescribe drugs and surgery to reverse what they diagnose as negative conditions. Certainly they know that diet and exercise matter and that negative buildup of stress takes a toll on the body. Most don't know what to recommend apart from a prescriptive and often addictive pill to reduce stress.

Very few physicians have time or inclination to keep up with the cutting edge of scientific research about how to stay healthy. Very few are willing—nor do they know how—to give you a detailed prescription for slowing the aging process or doing all you can to avoid arthritis, osteoporosis, lower-back pain, high blood pressure, coronary-artery disease, or ulcers. In summary, don't expect your personal family physician to be an expert these topics.

What your physician can do for you is to conduct very specific and beneficial blood tests to reveal your cholesterol level, hormone levels, and thyroid level. In addition, you'll get your weight from a doctor's scale and an accurate blood-pressure reading.

On your own, apart from your physician, you can complete the measurement portion of the following data sheet.

As you measure your waist—which is your girth at the level of your navel—do it two ways. First, pull your stomach in as far as you can, and measure. Then, let out your stomach and measure again. Record both measurements. Why? Because as you do tummy-flattening exercises, these measurements will be an effective means of recording your progress. Every month, remeasure. You'll see real differences starting in the second and third months.

PERSONAL DATA SHEET

DATE:

NAME:

WEIGHT (Update weekly.):

BLOOD PRESSURE (Update weekly, you can do this at home.):

BMI (Update monthly.):

BODY FAT PERCENTAGE (update monthly.):

CHOLESTEROL (Update annually unless it is high, then update quarterly.):

THYROID FUNCTION (It is only necessary to check once unless there is a problem.):

HORMONE LEVELS (testosterone in men, estrogen in women, Everyone should test levels of DHEA and Human growth hormone.):

(Note: if you do not want to test the levels of hormones and thyroid, make sure you take all other measurements.)

MEASUREMENTS (UPDATE MONTHLY):

NECK:

UPPER ARM:

ABOVE THE BUST/CHEST:

BUST/CHEST:

MIDWAY BETWEEN BUST/CHEST AND WAIST

WAIST (pulled in):

WAIST (let out):

ABDOMEN:

HIPS:

UPPER THIGH:

KNEE:

CALF:

ANKLE:

Check Your Own Thyroid Periodically.

You can also do the following to periodically check your thyroid function. Take your temperature upon awakening in the morning for four mornings in a row. The ideal range is between 97.8 and 98.2 degrees Fahrenheit. If you are a woman in child-bearing years, you will want to make sure you take your temperature for four days *after* a menstrual period has ended. That's the most accurate time in your monthly cycle for this reading. If your morning temperature is less than it was when you started your diet, your thyroid is now less active. When body temperature is reduced, low-calorie diets stop working. (There are several things you can do to jump-start a sluggish thyroid. See the chapter titled "The Supplements You Need to Fight the Fat War.")

Determine Your Ideal Body Weight.

What should your ideal weight be? That's a personal matter, but for most of the people I have counseled, ideal weight is usually their weight when they graduated from high school (assuming that they were not overweight in high school). A high school senior is generally fully developed and active enough to be fit.

For others, ideal weight is the amount they weighed when they married. Most people try to be trim and fit for their wedding and as they start their married life together.

Below are two tables to help you determine your ideal body weight. These tables have been put out by Metropolitan Life. They reflect the general standard adopted by most physicians. The weights listed are for ages twenty-five to fifty-nine.

Remember as you look at these numbers that if you work out with weights regularly and have increased your lean muscle weight, these charts may not be as accurate. That is why it is important to use a body fat caliper.

IDEAL BODY WEIGHT FOR MEN

Height In Feet/Inches	Small Frame	Medium Frame	Large Frame
5' 2"	125-131	128-138	135-148
5' 3"	127-133	130-140	137-151
5' 4"	129-135	132-143	139-155
5' 5"	131-137	134-146	141-159
5' 6"	133-140	137-149	144-163
5' 7"	135-143	140-152	147-167
5' 8"	137-146	143-155	150-171
5' 9"	139-149	146-158	153-175
5' 10"	141-152	149-165	156-179
5' 11"	144-155	155-169	159-183
6' 0"	147-159	159-173	163-187
6' 1"	150-163	162-177	167-192
6' 2"	153-163	166-182	171-197
6' 3"	157-167	170-187	176-202
6' 4"	161-171	171-187	181-207

IDEAL BODY WEIGHT FOR WOMEN

Height In Feet/Inches	Small Frame	Medium Frame	Large Frame
4'9"	99-108	106-118	115-128
4'10"	100-110	108-120	117-131
4'11"	101-112	110-123	119-134
5'0"	103-115	112-126	122-137
5'1"	105-118	115-129	125-140
5' 2"	108-121	118-132	128-144
5' 3"	111-124	121-135	131-148
5' 4"	114-127	124-138	134-152
5' 5"	117-130	127-141	137-156
5' 6"	120-133	130-144	140-160
5' 7"	123-136	133-147	143-164
5' 8"	126-139	136-150	146-167
5' 9"	129-142	139-153	149-170
5' 10"	132-145	142-156	152-173

Measure Your BMI Number.

Even more than weight, you should consider your BMI number. This measurement refers to Body Mass Index (BMI).

BMI is calculated as weight in kilograms divided by the square of the height in meters (kg/m^2). BMI is independent of age or sex although there are certain limitations to its use—BMI may not be the best index for children, pregnant women, or highly muscular individuals, such as athletes.

"Normal" for a person is determined by many physicians as comparing a person's ideal body weight and BMI. Those with a BMI of less than 27 are considered in the acceptable range, with a BMI of 20 to 25 being ideal. Mild obesity is defined as those with a body weight of 20 to 40 percent above the ideal body weight and a BMI of between 27 and 29. Moderate obesity is defined as 40 to 100 percent above ideal body weight and a BMI of between 30 and 40. Approximately four million Americans currently have BMIs between 35 and 40. Morbid obesity, also called clinically severe obesity, is defined as 100 percent or more above ideal body weight or a BMI above 40.

Here's how to use the following chart: Read down the column on the far left until you find your height in inches. Then read across that column until you find your weight. Then look back at the top of that column to find your Body Mass Index number. For example, a person who is 69 inches tall (5' 9") and weighs 216 has a BMI of 32.

BODY MASS INDEX FOR MEN AND WOMEN

The column to the far left is height in inches.
The numbers across the top of the chart are BMI numbers.

	18	19	20	21	22	23	24	25	26	27	28	29	30	31	**32**	33	34	35	36	37	38	39	40+
58	86	91	96	100	105	110	115	119	124	129	134	138	143	148	153	158	162	167	172	177	181	186	191+
59	89	94	99	104	109	114	119	124	128	133	138	143	148	153	158	163	168	173	178	183	188	193	198+
60	92	97	102	107	112	118	123	128	133	138	143	148	153	158	163	168	173	179	183	188	194	199	204+
61	95	100	106	111	116	122	127	132	137	143	148	153	158	164	169	174	180	186	191	195	201	206	211+
62	98	104	109	115	120	126	131	136	142	147	153	158	164	169	175	180	186	191	197	202	207	213	218+
63	101	107	113	118	124	130	135	141	146	152	158	163	169	175	180	186	191	197	203	208	214	220	225+
64	105	110	116	122	128	134	140	145	151	157	163	169	174	180	186	192	197	204	209	215	221	227	232+
65	108	114	120	126	132	138	144	150	156	162	168	174	180	186	192	198	204	210	216	222	228	234	240+
66	112	118	124	130	136	142	148	155	161	167	173	179	186	192	198	204	210	216	222	228	234	241	247+
67	115	121	127	134	140	146	153	159	166	172	178	185	191	198	204	211	217	223	230	236	242	249	255+
68	118	125	131	138	144	151	158	164	171	177	184	190	197	203	210	216	223	230	236	243	249	256	262+
69	122	128	135	142	149	155	162	169	176	182	189	196	203	209	**216**	223	232	236	243	250	257	263	270+
70	125	132	139	146	153	160	167	174	181	188	195	202	209	216	223	229	236	243	250	257	264	271	278+
71	129	136	143	150	157	165	172	179	186	193	200	208	215	222	229	236	243	250	257	265	272	279	286+
72	132	140	147	154	162	169	177	184	191	199	206	213	221	228	235	242	250	258	265	272	279	287	294+
73	140	147	154	161	168	176	182	189	197	204	212	219	227	234	242	250	257	265	272	280	287	295	303+
74	147	154	161	167	175	181	187	194	202	210	218	225	233	241	249	256	264	272	280	288	295	303	311+
75	154	161	167	175	181	187	193	200	208	216	224	232	240	247	255	263	271	279	287	295	303	311	319+
76	161	167	174	180	186	192	198	204	213	221	230	238	246	254	262	271	279	287	295	303	312	320	328+

GETTING ARMED FOR BATTLE!

Now that you have your "numbers" you should feel armed with the baseline information you need for taking action. Basically, you have "scouted" out your enemy.

The next step is to identify your "war goals" and to name the "spoils" that will go to the victor. That's where we turn next.

KEY #2:

Set realistic goals and motivating rewards.

4

SET A TARGET YOU CAN
AND *WANT* TO HIT

My buddy Zig Ziglar tells how he was overweight by more than forty pounds when he began to write his first book. He wrote his desired weight into the manuscript and that became his goal—he was determined to weigh that amount by the time he finished writing the manuscript! He set a reachable, realistic, but challenging goal.

Goals are tremendously important to a fat-loss plan. They are critical for success. Let me give you an example.

I am absolutely confident that within five minutes, I could have you shooting a bow and arrow better than the gold-medal winner in archery at the last Olympics competition.

When I make that statement to audiences they shake their heads and say, "How can you possibly do that?"

I respond, "We are going to blindfold the gold-medal winner. Then we are going to spin that person around twenty-five times and let him shoot at the target, wherever he thinks it may be."

That's silly, you may be thinking. Of course the gold-medal winner will fail miserably. Nobody can hit a target he can't see.

That is right. No one can hit a target they cannot see. If you do not set a target or a goal to accomplish for fat loss, there is no way to accomplish it. That is why goals are so critical to your ongoing success in all areas of your life.

DON'T JUST DREAM IT—*GOAL* IT!

There are countless motivational books on the market today and I have read many of them. One thing I've noticed about these books is that they make a very clear distinction between a person's *dreams* and a person's *goals*.

A dream is a vague whim or hope. "Someday I want to be thin" and "It sure would be nice to weigh less" and "I'm not always going to be so out of shape—someday I'll get back in shape" are dreams. They may or may not come to pass. In most cases they are snippets of wishful thinking.

A goal is something very specific that is set *into a time frame* and has a method for accomplishing the goal attached to it.

"Within ten weeks, I am going to lose ten pounds of fat and gain five pounds of muscle through eating properly and exercising daily." Now that's a *goal*. It's specific. It's got a time frame. It's got a method attached to it.

What is your goal for fat loss?

A Dose of Realism

There are several things that are vitally important for you to keep in mind as you set a fat-loss goal. That goal must take into consideration:

- your height

- your bone structure

- your age

Be ambitious but not ridiculous. Think attainable and doable. If you don't have any idea about what is realistic in fat loss, ask someone who has lost fat and maintained that loss for more than a year. I recommend not more than around two pounds of *weight* loss a week. If you are willing to work out every day, and to do so with intensity and diligence, you might gain a pound of muscle a month. That's going to be a net loss of seven pounds in a month.

The Basic Arithmetic

There's a basic arithmetic to fat loss. Every pound of body fat is equal to 3,500 calories. To lose one pound a week of body fat, you must burn up 3,500 calories *more* than you need to maintain your normal body function. To lose fat at a safe, even pace of two pounds a week, you need to burn up or reduce an additional 7,000 calories beyond what you would normally use.

Face the Fact that Your Obesity Didn't Happen Overnight.

I've already told one snake story but I'm going to tell another.

When I was twelve years old my family owned a fish camp. Beside the fish camp was a drainage canal that ran from Lake Mariana to Lake Jessie. Depending on the weather and the amount of rainfall we received, that canal could be dry or have up to three feet of water in it. The canal, of course, was prone to weed overgrowth and a considerable part of my responsibility in helping with the fish camp was to work with my mom to keep the weeds in that canal under control.

Florida has a great many mosquitoes and snakes and alligators. Alligators have even been found in suburban swimming pools. Water moccasins and rattlesnakes are also common predators in Florida. It was partly to keep the snakes away that we fought to keep the weeds in the canal under control.

One day when I had a shovel in my hand, I encountered a five-foot water moccasin, about four inches in diameter, swimming in the shallow waters of the canal close to where I was standing. These cottonmouth water moccasins are deadly, especially to children. I hit the water moccasin with the blunt end of the shovel, which only made it very mad. It came out of that water and landed on the bank close to me, trying to bite me. I probably moved as quickly as my wife did when she stepped on that other snake. We are both very blessed not to have been bitten.

Fat gain is not like a snakebite. It doesn't happen quickly or unexpectedly. Fat gain occurs over months and months and years and years.

If you put on only one pound of fat a month—that's only 3,500 extra calories, or only about 115 extra calories a day—you will gain twelve pounds in a year. Over a decade, you'll gain one hundred and twenty pounds! All from consuming only 115 extra calories a day beyond what your body needs.

You won't wake up one morning to discover that you have become obese overnight. You have gained the excess fat over time, and it's going to take some time for you to discard that fat. Don't expect an overnight drop of ten pounds, or even five pounds. Don't expect to lose all you've acquired in a month, or six months, if you are morbidly obese. Part of your challenge is going to be this: You must have patience with your own progress and continue to endure in your quest to lose excess fat.

A steady, even weight loss of a couple of pounds a week is much more healthful. In fact, the famous Framingham Heart Study (done over two decades) found that those whose weight changed a lot or changed often had a higher occurance of coronary heart disease. That's no excuse for remaining obese! It is a signal that you should count on losing fat slowly and evenly over several weeks, months, or even years.

Don't let these facts discourage you. Rather, consider them to be a dose of reality as you set a genuinely ambitious and challenging goal for yourself! And then . . .

WRITE DOWN YOUR GOAL

Almost fifty years ago, a Harvard University study showed that only 3 percent of the students who graduated that particular year had written down specific career goals. Twenty years later, a team of researchers interviewed the students who had participated in that original study. They found that the 3 percent who had written down their goals were worth more financially than the other 97 percent *combined*!

Those who write down their goals are far more motivated to pursue them, and to continue to pursue them until they reach them. In fact, research has shown that people who write down their goals are thirty times more likely to achieve them.

Write in Positive Terms.

Always write your fat-loss goals in positive terms. Use the phrase "I will!"

Don't write, "I hope to lose some weight."

Do write, "I *will* weigh 165 pounds and have less than 15 percent body fat by May 1."

Write in Personal Terms.

Use "I" when writing your goal. You'll be more motivated if you see yourself in your goal.

Give Yourself a Deadline.

Deadlines seem to have a built-in power to them. They boost motivation and increase results. When you set a deadline, you take a powerful mental steptoward making something happen. Your mind immediately begins to process the specific steps you must take to reach your goal. You will want to set two types of deadlines: ultimate and incremental.

For some people, an ultimate deadline might be linked to a longer-range goal such as a milestone event in your life—a major birthday, a charity walk, a hiking trip, an anniversary party, a child's wedding, a special vacation, a plan to meet a long-lost friend after ten years of not seeing each other.

I recommend that you post a picture that is related to your goal—perhaps a photo of the person you are planning to meet, the party invitation, a poster about the tournament or charity walk, a photo of the place you are planning to vacation in, or a photo of a birthday cake—where you can see it daily and where it will both remind and motivate you that "today's the day" for taking another step toward your ultimate desired destination.

If you're just coasting along in life, chances are you aren't really going anywhere. It's when you set a destination point that you tend to rev up the engines and map out a course of action. So use an ultimate goal to get started.

Several Incremental Deadlines. After you have set an ultimate deadline, set a deadline for reaching each very specific and short-term fat-loss goal. I recommend five-pound increments. In other words, mark a date on the calendar for losing five pounds of fat. When you reach your goal by that date, mark a date for losing another five pounds of fat.

If you are like most of my clients, you will probably find that a deadline in the very near future intensifies your resolve not to cheat in your eating and to maintain your exercise program. Your focus is maintained.

I suggest you purchase a calendar that is designated solely as your fat-loss calendar (or use the one provided in the *Maximum Fat Loss Workbook*).

Count the weeks between today's date and your goal date. At a rate of two pounds a week, how much fat can you reasonably expect to lose in that time frame? Based on the total, set incremental goals for each week, perhaps writing them in pencil onto your fat-loss calendar and then confirming them in ink when you have reached the mark. You can also use the same calendar to record the changes in you body fat percentages.

MAKE A PLAN FOR CHARTING YOUR PROGRESS

After you have broken down your goals into periodic checkpoints, weigh yourself once a week, at the same time each week. Friday mornings seem to be a good time for many people. Ideally you should weigh at home in the early morning on an accurate scale, with nothing on and before you have taken in *any* fluids or food.

I never recommend that a person get on the scales every day. Fluid weight in the body can vary up to two or more pounds in twenty-four hours, and a person can become greatly discouraged after two days of doing everything right, only to discover that the scales have gone *up* rather than down.

Remeasure your body measurements every month, on the same day of the month, for your overall progress.

Focus on your *progress* and the habits you're developing. That's far more important the first few months than the actual pounds lost or sizes reduced. The long-term patterns and habits are what will benefit you most when it comes to achieving maximum fat loss and maintaining that loss over the coming months and years.

A chart for monitoring your progress is included in the *Maximum Fat Loss Workbook.* I highly recommend that you buy this workbook—it's inexpensive and you'll find it an invaluable tool. If you can't find the workbook at your local bookstore, you can call my office: 1–800–726–1834.

DEVELOP A STRATEGY FOR OVERCOMING OBSTACLES

After you have written down your goals and broken them into specific sub-goals—all with deadlines—list three things you believe will prevent you from reaching your goal. For some it might be giving up a beloved snack food. I once heard about a woman who was willing to give any diet and exercise plan a try as long as she could keep eating all the potato chips and tortilla chips she wanted. It wasn't until I told her exactly how many fat grams were in ten regular potato chips that she said, "Well, I just might have to compromise a little here!"

For others, the obstacle that is likely to trip them up is not a food item but pressure from family members, close friends, or colleagues to engage in all-you-can-eat-until-you're-sick, pig-out feasts and lazy evenings in front of the television set. For still others the obstacle that impedes progress might be a work schedule that doesn't seem to leave a bit of room for a weight-training workout. (I promise you, if you really want to work out you'll find the time. I work out at home. You may very well find that over the coming months and year you will desire to develop a home gym in that spare bedroom that is rarely used!) This is why my basic exercise videos are done at home. They teach you exactly what to do in your home. It is also important for you to know that for every one pound of muscle you gain you actually increase your basic metabolic rate by fifty calories a day. The only way I know to increase muscle is resistance training.

If you set a goal and fail to pursue it or fail to endure until you reach it, don't worry about it. There's an old saying: "You're not out as long as you keep getting up every time you are knocked down." Take that thinking to heart. Simply refuse to give up in the pursuit of your fat-loss goals. Always see yourself as a winner, even though you may have experienced a temporary slipup.

A GOAL FOR YOUR MIND: A NEW OUTLOOK ON YOUR HEALTH

A person once said to me, "Starting a fat-loss program sounds as if I'm going to be adding a lot of pressure to my life."

On the one hand, she was correct. "Yes," I replied, "that's true. But a certain amount of pressure is good." Not all pressure or stress is necessarily negative. A certain amount of pressure is necessary for a person to feel excited and passionate about life. Many of the feats we call heroic are feats that are performed under pressure: a fireman rescuing a child from a burning building, a quarterback scoring the winning touchdown with thirty seconds on the clock, a surgeon performing an emergency procedure. Stress tends to be a very positive influence in reaching a goal on a timely manner!

Stress turns sour when we set *unreachable,* and therefore unrealistic, goals or deadlines. Don't set yourself up for failure by setting a goal to be gymnast-thin when you are thirty years old, five-feet-eight-inches tall, with a large bone structure! Don't envision yourself as a ballerina if you have butterfly-stroke swimmer's shoulders. And don't expect to lose a hundred pounds in three months! Working toward impossible goals can create negative stress in your body because you are working toward something that simply cannot be accomplished.

Most overweight people have *too little pressure* in their lives when it comes to losing fat, and too much pressure in other areas. Those areas may be work, family problems, or inner emotional problems. Cut out the negative stress in the nonphysical areas of your life and you'll have plenty of room for accommodating any physical pressure that a fat-loss program might create.

I once knew a fifty-year-old couch potato. He loved a good party and a life of ease. But then he took a truly objective look at his body and his life and decided that his life had ceased to become satisfying and he had no great sense of either purpose or fulfillment. He also took an objective look in the mirror and realized that he didn't like the "fat old man" staring back at him. He said to himself, *That's not the real me,* and he set out to unleash the person hiding behind all that fat. He determined that he was going to lose his excess fat and reshape his body and his life . . . and he made that determination with a do-or-die intent. He literally said, "I'm going to do this or they'll find me dead in the gym!" The fact was he honestly believed that if he didn't lose the excess fat and change some things in his life, he would die prematurely.

Did this man put himself under pressure? Yes. But it was positive pressure. He set goals and rewards and interim deadlines and began a strict program. He later told me that the program required more self-discipline and greater time management than anything else he had ever done. But one hundred and forty-two days later he had lost fifty pounds. He had muscles where he hadn't seen muscles in a very long time. And he found that his life changed completely—not only did his appearance change, but his optimism level began to soar, he began to set new goals in other areas of his life, he felt much greater energy, he was much quicker to spend time with friends, he had a completely different outlook on the purpose for his life, and he had a much different perspective on what he needed to do to feel fulfilled on any given day.

Is he an unusual case? Far from it. He's the norm for those who truly focus on a fat-loss program and decide to take charge of their own health and well-being.

Set your mind on developing new habits, not on a daily "reading of the scale."

A NEW COMMITMENT OF YOUR WILL

Goals are one thing. A commitment to reaching your goals is another. Just as a decision needs to be turned into a desire, a goal needs to be sealed with a commitment.

I recommend that you make a contract with yourself as a statement of your commitment. Here's a sample:

MY CONTRACT FOR IMPROVING MY HEALTH

I will work to attain a healthy, lean body.

I will adopt quality health habits—spiritual, physical and emotional habits that build genuine wholeness—as the foundation for living quality life.

I deeply desire to make this commitment and I will do all I can to improve my health and accomplish my fat-loss goals:

- I choose to eat the things that I know are right for good health.

- I will exercise regularly.
- I will drink sufficient water and take into my body both sufficient fiber and nutrients (including high-quality supplements).
- I will focus on what is good for me rather than give in to what is bad for me.
- I will be grateful for each day's blessings, including the blessing of improving health.

If I do not succeed at the rate I had hoped, I will reexamine what I am doing, make any necessary adjustments, and choose to persevere in my fat-loss program.

If I miss a goal at any point, I will consider it nothing but a temporary setback and a learning experience and I will try again.

I will reward myself for the fat I lose at incremental levels.

I will choose to think well of myself and to see myself as lean and thin regardless of what a scale may say or how I may feel emotionally on any given day.

Signed:_____

Date:_____

A TRUE COMMITMENT CREATES ENERGIZING POWER

Do you remember the first time you experienced a truly significant event in your life? I call these *power moments.* They are moments that not only give us a reason for getting up in the morning, but compel us to action and to giving our all every hour of every day. They are moments that make us feel fully alive! Maybe it was the day you graduated, the day your children were born, or the day you experienced a spiritual epiphany. Maybe it was the time when you first knew you were in love and that you wanted to marry the person who had captured your heart. Take a moment to recall one of those power moments in your life.

That's the way I hope you will feel when you make a firm commitment to pursue and then maintain a fat-loss program. Turning away from excess fat and ill health, and toward a lean, healthy body is a major moment.

A PLAN FOR REWARDING YOURSELF

No set of goals is complete without a plan for rewarding yourself for reaching both your ultimate goal and your incremental sub-goals.

Rewards are what add a dimension of motivation to any fat-loss plan. They are the pat on the back that makes all of your hard work and diligence worthwhile.

Some of the rewards are virtually automatic—such as better health, more energy, less pain, greater flexibility, higher self-esteem, increased sociability, and ambition.

Other rewards should be tangible. You eventually will be able to *see* your weight loss. However, tangible rewards that you can see, touch, and experience can help you through those times when you know good things are happening to your body *internally, but* until you have no external evidence. Tangible rewards are especially important for those who have forty or more pounds to lose. The first few pounds may not be all that noticeable to you or to others. A tangible reward can help you stay on track—it serves as a reminder that you are making good progress.

Whatever the rewards you establish for yourself as part of your fat-loss goals, they should be big enough to create deep within you an intense desire to reach your goal. If your rewards don't motivate you toward positive achievement, set different rewards or aim at a higher goal. Donald Trump once said, "If you're going to be thinking anyway, you might as well think big!" I agree. Set some powerful, grand goals for yourself. And then attach some significant rewards to them!

Rewards Are Highly Personal.

What is rewarding to you may not be at all rewarding to the next person. In the end, what you choose as a reward and what you find rewarding are strictly up to you. Don't ever think to yourself, *It's silly to think of rewarding myself in this way.* YOU are the main reason for you to lose fat. It's your body, your health, your appearance. And in the end, it's up to you to motivate yourself toward reaching the goals you set. Your rewards are *your* rewards.

You may not be wise to share with others your goals or the rewards you plan to give to yourself. In many cases that only makes you subject to their nagging, teasing, or even criticism. Only share your goals with those who are supportive of both your efforts to lose fat and to reward yourself in the ways you choose.

Be very careful that you don't reward yourself with food, including an expensive or luxurious meal out. Choose nonfood rewards! Consider instead the reward of a night out at the theater (without dinner), a vacation, workout equipment, a cardio machine, a new work-out outfit, a new accessory, and for you ladies, even a luxurious half-day to yourself to pamper your body with a manicure, pedicure, facial, and long, soaking bubble bath!

Treat Yourself to a Monthly Massage.

One of the nicest ways you can reward yourself is also a therapeutic way to help yourself in the fat-loss process.

A massage is not just a luxury. Massage can have a number of health-related benefits, especially to the person who is pursuing a fat-loss program.

A massage can help muscles that are weary or over-exercised to heal faster. Massage greatly helps healing of strains in muscles and connective tissue, spasms and pain that restrict movement, edema and swelling, and metabolic waste buildup that causes muscle fatigue.

Massage can help you stay flexible because pressure, stretching, and friction all raise the temperature of your tissues. Even a slight increase in the temperature of your muscles promotes more fluid within the tissues and this helps reduce rigidity, eliminate waste, and promotes the transport of nutrients into the muscles so you can move without pain.[1]

Massage has mental effects apart from just plain ol' feeling good. Studies have shown that massage releases hormones that can speed healing, ease pain, and help clear the mind. In one study done with premature babies, the babies who were massaged were more alert, slept better, and scored higher on both mental and motor tests.[2]

A massage also can help break down the small fibrous networks of tissue that sometimes tend to freeze muscles or trap fat.

Are you aware that in international athletic competition, a massage therapist is considered on par with medical doctors, physical therapists, osteopaths, nurses, and athletic trainers as part of many a national team's medical support staff? In 1996 massage was officially included at the Atlanta Olympic games as part of the medical team's services.

How often should you get a massage? Many professional athletes see a massage therapist twice a week. For most people, a visit once every three to four weeks is more normal. Be sure to go to a licensed massage therapist. And try to schedule your visit after you've had a good vigorous workout. You'll experience even greater benefits.

Start a New-Clothes Fund.

Another tangible and beneficial way many women and some men reward themselves is with "gifts" of their own money. Get out the old piggy bank and put a twenty dollar bill into it every time you lose a pound. The reality is this: You are going to need some new clothes, or alterations to your old ones, as you lose weight. That's a joyful prospect for most people. Have fun spending your money as you buy clothes in a smaller size!

TAKE AN IMMEDIATE ACTION STEP . . . TODAY!

Don't put off acting on your goals. The worst thing a good goal can do is gather dust in a notebook. Start realizing your goals. Take a positive step toward your first reward!

Nearly all people who start a fat-loss program will need to do three things:

Schedule Your New Regimen.

Write your new pattern of action onto your calendar—*in detail.* Schedule your meals and workout sessions and write down when you intend to *take* your supplements. (More on these topics later.) Make a check-off place for drinking sufficient water. (A full daily schedule is offered in the *Maximum Fat Loss Workbook.*)

Plan Your Eating for a Week.

Plan out a week's worth of meals and an accompanying grocery list. Also, you can freeze meals to make them more convenient. To make this easier order my wife's cookbook from my office. [4]

Redo the Contents of Your Pantry

Stock up the groceries you need and at the same time eliminate from your cupboards all the foods that you know are counter-productive to your weight-loss plan. Take the unopened products back to the grocery store for a refund. Or you can give the items to a needy cause. By eliminate, I do not mean eat! You may feel "bad" throwing out half a bag of potato chips or tossing a couple of cans of sugar-filled soda. Do it anyway. Promise yourself you won't waste food in the future by also promising yourself that you won't buy junk foods in the first place! Then . . .

List any other things you need to do to put in place your new plan for losing weight. Here are some of the most common things I have found among my clients:

- Join a gym to have access to weight-training equipment.

- Get a pair of good walking shoes (primarily for use on the nonimpact cardiovascular equipment available at better gyms).

- Go to the local health food store and purchase the supplements necessary to enhance a fat-loss program. If you are unable to find these items call my office. My trained staff will be happy to assist you.

You'll find other things as you work your way through the remaining chapters of this book. Write them down as you go.

One note: I strongly recommend that you try a type of exercise for awhile before you purchase any home equipment. Don't put "buy a treadmill" or "buy a home gym set" or "build a swimming pool" on your list! Wait until you are fully into an exercise routine before you make investments of that magnitude.

You may, however, want to obtain a copy of my *Forever Fit* tape series or, as I mentioned earlier, order a set of my exercise videos. Perhaps you need a personal trainer. You may also want to list "join a weight-loss support group" (or even better, "join a *fat*-loss support group").[5]

Do something *today* to send a signal to your mind and your heart that you are serious about pursuing your goals.

And now, get ready for the nitty-gritty: of the behaviors you actually need to adopt to implement an effective fat-loss program.

KEY #3:

Eat six meals a day, with a calorie total not exceeding ten times your ideal body weight.

5

FEED YOUR BODY
OFTEN AND WELL

If you want to lose weight, simply burn more calories than you consume." Most people who undertake a weight-loss or fat-loss program have heard that statement more times than they can count. Taken word for word, it's a true statement. But this statement is definitely outdated, incomplete, and vague when it comes to the most recent research in physiology and biochemistry.

Let me help you get up-to-date as quickly and simply as possible.

First, as we have already covered, to lose *weight* is not the true goal. *Fat* loss is the goal. When it comes to fat loss, not all calories are created equal.

Second, meal timing, food selection, and the types and timing of exercise are also as important to fat loss as the number of calories a person eats. Scientific evidence also shows that supplementation of nutrients can help. (We will address exercise and supplements later in this book.)

Now, given those two statements, you might assume that I will tell you that you don't need to count calories. Initially, until you get used to portion sizes, you will need to deal with a calorie *total* per day. Which foods are best for you to choose in reaching that calorie total is another issue. So is when you eat the calories and how you exercise them away. A total daily calorie count, nevertheless, is important to getting started on a fat-loss program.

HOW MANY CALORIES SHOULD YOU CONSUME?

Your total calorie count is based on what you *want* to weigh, not on what you presently weigh. Multiply your ideal weight by ten.

Let me give you an example. Let's suppose you are a woman and you want to weigh 120 pounds. Take your ideal weight (120) and multiply it by 10. Result: 1,200. That's the number of calories you should consume per day to reach your ideal weight and stay there. Never go *under* this amount.

Another example: If you are a man who desires to weigh 180 pounds, you will need to consume 1,800 calories a day.

Eat six meals a day.

Once you have determined your total calorie count for a day, divide that number by six. This gives you the average number of calories for each meal of your day.

For the woman who wants to weigh 120 pounds and who has a total calorie count of 1,200 calories a day, each meal will be 200 calories.

For the man who wants to weight 180 pounds and who has a total calorie count of 1,800 calories a day, each meal will be 300 calories.

"Whoa, Ted," I can hear you saying. "That's not many calories." The challenge is: Most of us need a new definition of "a healthy meal."

Redefine "a healthy meal" for yourself.

"Eat six healthy meals a day" sounds like fairly straightforward advice. But I have discovered through the years that most people do not have a good definition of "healthy"! A meal with an appetizer, dessert, bread and butter, four side dishes, and a soft drink alongside the main entrée is not a healthy meal.

A healthy meal is one that totals only a few hundred calories, usually between two hundred and three hundred calories.

How do you know what totals two-to three hundred calories in a healthy meal? Initially, you are going to have to count calories and evaluate portion size.

I'm not high on calorie counting except at the *outset* of a person's move toward maximum fat loss. Over time, the general calorie intake is going to be ingrained in your mind and you won't need to count calories. At the outset, however, a person needs to count calories for one main reason: Most people do not know the caloric value of foods.Therefore they have no concept as to how much they can eat of certain foods and still consume only two hundred to three hundred calories per meal. People tend to be shocked when I point out that a pat of butter contains one hundred calories—and two or three pats of butter is not a good healthy meal!

To help you count calories, purchase a very simple calorie counter. A number of them are on the market, from printed lists to electronic calculating devices. Choose a counter you will carry and use. (Or, you can consult the calorie counter in the *Maximum Fat Loss Workbook.*)

No fudging.

There are two ways people tend to fudge on their calorie counting and I think we need to face these head-on:

1. *Lean meat is* lean *meat.* Calorie counters give a count for lean meat. Make sure all fat is trimmed away from your meat sources—skin from chicken, fat from beef. If you are eating chopped meat, choose ground round steak rather than ground hamburger because it is leaner. Don't eat pork or fatty fish (such as mackerel). Stay with bass, grouper, snapper, or whiting.

2. *Ounces* are measurable ounces. Most people do not have a

good idea at the outset of a fat-loss program as to how much an item weighs by merely looking at it. To determine how much a meat or vegetable portion weighs, you are going to have to put it on a scale. If you don't have a reliable food scale, purchase one. It's a worthy investment.

Deal in actual weight of items. Scoops vary in size, as any child can tell you when it comes to scoops on an ice cream cone! The size of a "spoonful," "portion," or the number of ounces in a "small size" can also vary greatly.

Keep track of your calories. Initially, keeping a food journal is a simple way to register what you eat and the calorie count for each food. Keep in mind that you must write down *every* item of food or nonwater beverage that you consume in a day, including a mint or an extra celery stick.

You might want to use a check-register pad for your food journal. Give yourself an opening "balance" for the day, which is your total calorie count for that day. Use the "deposit" column for recording fat gram amounts and the balance column for your calories. Once you have consumed your total of fat grams, refuse to eat more fat. Subtract the calorie amounts as you move through the day. When you run out of calories, stop eating for the day! With proper planning, this won't happen until you have finished your last healthy meal of the day.

After several days or weeks of calculating calories, you are probably going to be able to judge the number of calories you are eating by the portion size of your protein foods and carbohydrates. A portion of food is roughly equal to the size of a clenched fist or the palm of your hand. A typical portion of protein contains between 100 and 150 calories (such as a chicken breast or small fillet of baked fish).

Have a healthy breakfast.

Most fat-loss experts agree that your highest nutrient density meal should come in the morning. Any big meal should be eaten after a workout. Ideally, your biggest meal should be breakfast, eaten after your morning cardiovascular workout. I personally consume a delicious meal- replacement shake after I work out. I'll provide the recipe in an upcoming chapter.

Big meal versus *small meal* doesn't mean a great deal, of course, in terms of overall calorie differences. If you are consuming an average of three hundred calories per meal, you might eat four hundred calories at your first meal of the day and only two hundred at your last meal. Most of your calories for each of these meals—first and last of the day—should be approximately 30 to 40 percent lean protein.

Be sure to finish your last meal of the day at least three hours before bedtime. If you must snack before bed, eat lean protein only.

Try incremental "step-down" calorie counting.

If you have a great deal of weight to lose—forty or more pounds—then you are likely to find that moving directly to the calorie count of your "ideal weight" is too difficult. An incremental step-down program is better suited for you.

Identify what you would weigh if you lost thirty pounds. How many calories should you consume at that weight? Multiply your weight by ten. Divide that weight by six for your average calorie count per meal.

Adjust your step-down program after you have lost ten pounds. Again, identify what you would weigh if you lost thirty pounds. Recalculate. Eventually you'll reach the week in which you are actually calculating the count for the final thirty pounds. (That's another good reward point!)

There's another way you can approach the step-down process. Subtract 500 calories from the number of calories you need to maintain your present weight. For example, if you weigh 300 pounds, to maintain your weight would require a 3,000-calorie day. Choose instead to consume 2,500 calories, or about 420 calories average for each of six small meals. Since one pound equals 3,500 calories, you can expect to lose a pound a week at that rate. (500 calories x 7 days = 3,500, which is the number of calories in a pound)

By implementing an exercise program to go along with your five hundred-fewer-calories-a-day plan (including all three forms of exercise outlined in a later chapter in this book) you will typically lose one to two pounds a week in fat while maintaining or even gaining muscle mass.[1]

EVENLY SPACE YOUR SIX MEALS

One of the easiest ways to space out these six meals is to eat three of the meals at regular mealtimes. Then space your snacks evenly between breakfast and lunch, lunch and early dinner, and between early dinner and bedtime. Ideally, you will be eating *something* nutritious every two-and-a-half waking hours. Here's a typical schedule:

Breakfast	7:00 A.M. (after aerobic
and	resistance exercise)
Midmorning snack	9:30 A.M.
Lunch	12:00 P.M.
Midafternoon snack	2:30 P.M.
Early dinner or late-afternoon snack	5:00 P.M.
Late dinner or evening snack	7:30 P.M.

SAMPLE MEALS

You may think you can't get much in the way of nutrients in a meal that has only two hundred to three hundred calories. To the contrary! Here are twenty-nine examples of two hundred to three hundred calorie meals.

- six egg whites and a small bowl of oatmeal with nonfat milk

- three ounces of skinless chicken and one cup low-glycemic-index vegetables

- three ounces of fish and one cup low-glycemic index vegetables

- a slice of skinless turkey breast with a handful of air-popped popcorn

- one cup of tomato dill soup with an open-face albacore tuna salad sandwich on a slice of whole-grain rye bread

- one cup of low-salt onion soup and a spinach salad topped with a few slices of red onion and the sections of an orange

- two cups of Chinese vegetables stir-fried with three ounces of chicken

- a three-ounce turkey burger on one half of a whole-wheat bun with slices of tomato, onion, and lettuce

- a broiled tomato served with four ounces of broiled fish and a cup of steamed greens (such as chard)

- a two-egg (whole egg or substitute) omelet with two ounces of nonfat cheese or cottage cheese and one-and-a half-cups of mixed tomatoes and chopped green peppers

- two cups of mixed-green salads with nonfat dressing; a half cup of vegetable broth; one and a half cups of steamed broccoli, red
peppers, onion, mushrooms, and zucchini topped with two ounces of plain nonfat yogurt; and a half cup of all-natural, sugar-free applesauce

- a cup of vegetable soup; a lettuce salad topped with sautéed pea pods, mushrooms, and asparagus; and three ounces of lean beef

- a cup of cooked oatmeal topped with a cup of plain, fat-free yogurt and a cup of strawberries

- a spinach salad; a cup of broccoli, peppers, onions, and mushrooms topped by a half cup of marinara sauce; and a half
cup of fat-free cottage cheese

- a four-ounce fish fillet, baked or poached; a cup of asparagus; a cup of zucchini; and a mixed salad with nonfat dressing

- two ounces of nonfat cottage cheese topped with several dashes of cinnamon; a half of a grapefruit; and half of a toasted whole-wheat bagel (no butter or cream cheese)

- half of a medium size papaya stuffed with a tuna salad made with nonfat plain yogurt, celery, and a few raisins and walnuts

- four ounces of roast lamb with a half cup each of fresh spinach and mushrooms

- eight ounces of nonfat milk, a cup of blueberries, and a cup of whole-grain cereal

- half a whole-wheat pita bread round stuffed with two scrambled eggs, chopped tomato and green pepper pieces, and an apple

- four ounces of turkey breast, one-and-a-half cups of steamed green beans, and a large mixed green salad with nonfat dressing

- two links of turkey sausage (no nitrite, well-drained), two scrambled eggs, and several slices of tomato and onions

- a cup of vegetarian chili, a slice of whole-grain bread, and a mixed green salad with nonfat dressing

- a cup of plain nonfat yogurt, a quarter cup of wheat germ, and half of a grapefruit

- three ounces of chicken breast, a cup of collard greens steamed with onions, and a cup of steamed zucchini

- two eggs scrambled with one ounce of smoked salmon, topped with a little chopped onion and a half teaspoon of capers, and served with a sliced tomato

- twelve ounces of hearty vegetable soup (preferably home-made—watch the sodium content on packaged mixes and canned soups)

- half of an avocado with two ounces of albacore tuna

- half of a pear and a half cup of cottage cheese

WHY DO THIS?

Eating six healthy meals throughout the day keeps your body from feeling the "starvation" effects associated with many weight-loss plans—those effects that often make a dieter feel grumpy and mentally foggy. By feeding your body throughout the day, you avoid hunger cramps and intense cravings and maintain a stable energy level.

From a physiological standpoint, six meals a day allows your blood-sugar levels and energy levels to be maintained, and the maximum percentage of nutrients to be absorbed by the body. The steady flow of amino acids and glucose feeds muscle tissue and helps your body maintain a healthy metabolism. Dr. Jeff Stout, a professor of exercise science at Creighton University, has called six-meals-a-day a "metabolic environment custom tailored to fat loss and muscle growth."[2]

Six meals a day is a means of addressing head-on the important hormone issue that underlies all fat gain and loss.

A QUICK CALORIE OVERVIEW

Below are several groups of food arranged according to calorie count:

I. One cup has an average of 35 calories

asparagus	cucumber
green beans	eggplant
broccoli	lettuce
cabbage	mushrooms
cauliflower	green peppers
celery	radishes

II. One cup has an average of 45 calories

artichoke	rutabagas
bean sprouts	turnips
beets	Brussels sprouts
carrots	peas
lima beans	squash

III. Average of 75 calories in serving sizes shown

cooked whole-grain cereal (½ cup)	unbuttered popcorn (1 ½ cups)
granola or whole-grain dry cereal (½ cup)	

IV. Average of 85 calories in serving sizes shown

avocado (½ cup)	nonfat milk (1 cup)
unflavored yogurt (½ cup)	

V. An average of 150 calories for two ounces

beef	turkey
lamb	fish
chicken	cottage cheese
eggs	

ADDRESSING THE CORE ISSUE: HORMONES AT WORK

I'm about to embark into an area that may leave you saying, "Hey, Ted. Just tell me how to drive the car. I don't need to know how the engine works."

I want you to know, however, a little about how the engine of your body works. I have found through many years of consulting with my clients that the more they know why they should do certain things related to fat loss, the more eager they are to do them and keep doing them. People have constantly written to me to tell me how much easier it is to say no to certain foods after they have ordered my *Eat, Drink and Be Healthy* program in which I explain why we shouldn't eat them. I certainly am not asking you to earn a doctorate in physiology or become an expert in this area. I want you to know what works and what doesn't and why.

One of the things that doesn't work is a high-carb, low-fat diet. And the reason it doesn't work is *hormonal*.

An alarm was sounded in the 1980s regarding the hazards of consuming too much dietary fat. Health experts warned against eating red meat, egg yolks, and poultry skin, and began to tout the virtues of a low-fat, high-carbohydrate diet. The promise was held out that such a diet would cause great weight loss without much pain. Food manufacturers got on the band wagon and began to introduce low-fat and fat-free products.

As it turns out, these very sincere health experts were sincerely wrong. A high-carbohydrate, low-fat diet actually makes matters worse!

The startling fact is that in the eleven years after the low-fat, high-carbohydrate diet campaign was launched in America, the number of Americans classified as obese rose from twenty-five percent to thirty-two percent! Our nation did not become thinner in the wake of a low-fat, high-carb craze, it became more obese!

Interestingly enough, the current food pyramid approved by the federal government reflects approximately the same protein, carbohydrate, and fat ratios as a sack of swine-fattening feed at your local farm and garden store. So unless you and your family are swine being fattened to go to market, why in the world would you want to eat this way? Of course even swine if told the end result, would probably choose another option. Let's face it, the market is a very negative experience for swine.

How can it be that we are dieting more and losing less? A low-fat, high-carb diet does not address the *hormonal* functions of insulin and glucagon.

For years, my office was deluged with telephone calls from people who wanted to know how they could lose weight and keep it off. Most of those who called admitted they had tried one or more diet plans with very little success.

Then I had a serious dose of personal experience with all this.

For the first twenty years that I worked in the field of health and nutrition, I maintained a diligent and disciplined personal exercise program. When I went on speaking tours I usually added a few pounds because my exercise regimen and food intake was interrupted, but when I returned to my normal schedule I was able to work off the extra pounds after a week or two in the gym.

Then I turned forty and things changed dramatically. I still put on those two or three pounds during an extended trip. My workouts after a trip were effective in eliminating the first pound quickly, but those last two pounds stubbornly refused to leave. I carried them with me into the next tour. Over the months, two stubborn pounds were added to two stubborn pounds to two stubborn pounds, and for the first time in many years I had a weight problem myself!

Now I was exercising just as strenuously as before but the extra weight clung to me like polyester pants filled with static electricity.

What did I do? I took the commonly accepted advice of the general scientific community and radically reduced my dietary fat intake. And I mean radically. The end result was that I consumed too little fat. My body couldn't produce enough essential fatty acids to nourish my skin and it became dry and flaky. Not only that; I didn't lose much weight! I gained an entirely new and personal understanding of the mental anguish experienced by those who battle chronic weight problems.

I spent several weeks pouring over the current scientific literature on diet and the human biochemical relationships between diet and weight gain. The question that haunted me was this: *Is there something wrong with my body or my metabolism?* The conclusion I reached was simply that the problem was hormonal.

The Hormonal Keys to Fat Loss

When most of us think of hormones, we tend to think of estrogen and testosterone, the most prominent sexual hormones for women and men. The fact is, however, that hormones regulate all bodily functions, including the key nutritional processes in the body such as blood sugar levels and fat storage.

Very specifically, the hormone that regulates the overall metabolism of the body is thyroid. Antidiuretic hormones regulate the water balance of the body through the kidneys. Insulin and glucagon regulate the metabolism of food, specifically glucose, and the burning of fat. These two hormones, insulin and glucagon, are the two key hormones responsible for fat gain and a difficulty in losing fat.

The real secret, therefore, in maintaining muscle mass and losing unhealthy body fat is learning how to control hormone level, and increase your basal metabolic rate. This becomes especially important as a person ages. Various hormone levels in the body change with age, and hormonal imbalance can cause numerous symptoms in the body—most of which are unpleasant—from increased fat storage to hot flashes.

Insulin and Glucagon—a Delicate Balance

Both insulin and glucagon are manufactured and released into the blood stream by the pancreas. Exercise and diet play a vital role in maintaining the balance of these hormones in the body.

Insulin is secreted into the system after we eat as a response to rising levels of sugars in the bloodstream. After a meal is consumed, the food is broken down into protein, fat, and carbohydrates. As the carbohydrates are digested, they are broken down further into glucose or sugar, the body's main fuel source. It is glucose that brings nourishment to all the cells of the body as it travels through the bloodstream. Not only is glucose the main fuel source for the body, it is the *only* fuel source for the brain.

Glucose, however, cannot enter a cell directly on its own. Glucose molecules are large molecules and they are kept out of cells by the fairly dense cell walls. It is insulin that works like a crowbar to pry open the cellular gateways to allow glucose to enter and bring nourishment to a cell.

Insulin is also responsible for reducing the levels of glucose in the bloodstream after the consumption of sugary meals. Under normal circumstances, when a person eats an extra serving of dessert with ice cream, his blood sugar level can rise to dangerously high levels in a matter of minutes. The pancreas secretes insulin to lower these sugar levels immediately by forcing glucose into body cells. (In diabetics, the pancreas no longer functions to secrete necessary amounts of insulin necessary for controlling sugar levels. This is why diabetics must receive injections of insulin to control their blood sugar levels.)

The key to weight gain, exercise, and insulin is found in yet another function of insulin: Insulin is a "storage hormone" that causes the body to store fuel for later use. It is the storage of excess glucose that is the root cause of virtually all weight problems.

Furthermore, insulin not only causes the storage of glucose as fat, but it blocks the body's ability to break down fat and burn it off. Too much insulin also inhibits the enzymes that promote fat oxidation and increases the activity of other enzymes that promote body fat accumulation.[3] Insulin secretion actually seems to be highest during sleep, so eating carbohydrates at bedtime is *especially* counterproductive to fat loss.[4] We can readily conclude that insulin is the villain in fat-loss metabolism.

The body has a limited capacity for storing glucose in its purest form. The purest form of instantly available stored glucose is *glycogen*, which is found almost exclusively in the liver and muscle tissues. Only about four hundred grams (sixteen hundred calories) of glucose can be stored in the body at any one time. The liver holds about one hundred grams and the muscles about three hundred grams.

Let me give you some perspective on this. Sixteen hundred calories is not a lot of extra fuel. If you stopped eating completely for some reason, this reserve of sixteen hundred calories could become depleted after only about thirty to ninety minutes of intense exercise. You may assume that it would be easy to replenish such a small "fuel tank," and this is a correct assumption. Sixteen hundred calories can be acquired with only one high-carbohydrate meal after intense exercise.

The problem is not, however, with depletion of the glycogen levels. The problem is that the vast majority of Americans consume way too many carbohydrates at every meal and have way too much glucose in their systems. The pancreas counters this excessive glucose with a major shot of insulin.

Glucose must be handled in one of three ways:

1. *Used for energy immediately* (and only so much can be forced into the body's cells and used at any given time).

2. *Stored as glycogen in the liver or muscle tissues* (although only four hundred grams total can be stored, and usually those storage tanks in the liver and muscles are filled). Muscle tissue is crucial in helping balance blood sugar levels. Under normal circumstances, more than 80 percent of the blood sugar released immediately following a meal is taken up by muscle cells. That's one of the reasons

that muscle-building exercise is so important. The greater your muscle mass, the more grams of glycogen you can store in muscle. If muscle cells become less sensitive to available insulin, the muscle cells cannot take up the influx of blood sugar after a meal. This insensitivity is also addressed in a later chapter and is an important issue.

3. *Stored as body fat* (the usual route). After the immediate energy needs of the body are met and all the fat possible has been stored in the liver and muscles, the body begins to store fat in its thirty-to forty billion fat cells. If the muscle and liver glycogen tanks are full, the glucose has no choice but to be turned into body fat.

What happened when I jumped on the high-carb, low-fat diet bandwagon? Every time I ate a fat-free, high-carb meal, my body responded to the high levels of glucose-producing carbohydrates in my bloodstream by releasing a large amount of insulin. This forced the overdose of glucose in my body cells. The excess glucose had to go somewhere. Some of it I burned up as energy during my workouts at the gym, but I could only burn so much at one time. Some of it was stored as glycogen to replenish my four-hundred-gram fuel tanks. Most of it, however, was converted to fat for storage. It was only when I began to reduce the amount of high-glycemic carbohydrates at mealtimes that my excess pounds came off and stayed off.

Stay with me because we're getting close to the heart of the matter regarding maximum fat loss!

There are two essential fat-loss facts you need to know:

1. *After glucose has been converted to fat, it can* not *be converted back to glucose.* Fat cannot be converted to sugar or muscle. The only practical way to get rid of fat is to burn it off through—you've guessed it—consistent aerobic or strength-building exercise.

2. *Protein* can *be converted to glucose.* Since glucose is needed as fuel for the brain, any time the body is deprived of food—such as during a fad diet—the body begins to scavenge for nutrients. After depleting all glycogen from the muscles and liver, it will go to stored *protein* to convert it to glucose. (The body does not go to stored fat

because fat cannot be converted back to glucose.) The result can be a radical loss of lean muscle mass. Once again, remember: For every pound of muscle you lose your basal metabolic rate is lowered by fifty calories per day.

Not too long ago I heard the story of a young woman who had decided that a no-fat, high-carb diet was the way to go. She jogged several miles a day to aid in her quest for a lean body. The result was not at all what she desired. The high-carb, no-fat diet forced her body to seek out protein for conversion to glucose and although she did lose some weight, she also lost a great deal of muscle weight. The muscles in her arms and legs atrophied and the result was far from flattering. Muscle loss and a slower metabolism are what tend to happen when the body begins to feed upon its muscle protein stores for glucose.

The Hero in this Hormone Saga

As noted earlier, insulin is the villain in battle of the bulge. Is there a superhero hormone? Absolutely. It's name is glucagon. I realize that glucose, glycogen, and glucagon are very similar words, and a person can easily become confused. If you are going to remember one word, remember the hero word: glucagon.

There is one other point about blood sugar levels and insulin I need to make. Whenever you elevate blood sugar quickly by eating refined or processed carbohydrates or even eating high glycemic carbohydrates (by the way, a baked potato will elevate blood sugar faster than table sugar) the body responds by increasing the insulin levels released by the pancreas. I have already explained that to you, but what I have not yet told you is equally as important. When we constantly elevate blood sugar and then drop it quickly, in some cases our bodies develop hypoglycemia. Hypoglycemia is the development of chronic low blood sugar. The symptoms include fatigue, dizziness, headache, irritability, bad temper, crying spells, depression, anxiety, craving for sweets, confusion, and mental disturbances.

Hypoglycemia is often misdiagnosed as Attention Deficit Disorder, Attention Deficit Disorder with hyperactivity, and in some cases even mental illness. I have found in my practice that many marriages have crumbled because of spouses with this condition.

So, your next question may be "Why are we discussing hypoglycemia in a fat-loss book?" The answer is actually very simple. When you have constant blood sugar drops due to insulin release, your body craves glucose. Remember, the brain must have available glucose at all times. When this occurs we have a constant craving for sweets.

Let me give you a real-world example. Several years ago a lady came in my office. I'll call her Sue. Sue was terribly hypoglycemic. She had lived on high-glycemic junk foods for years. For breakfast every morning she would eat a sugar-filled cereal, and by 10:00 A.M. her blood sugar had crashed and she was craving a sweet snack. By noon her snack had caused her sugar to crash again, causing her to crave more sweets. She had already gone through two marriages and was constantly juggling her mood swings and weight gain.

I call the situation that Sue had gotten herself into the "carbohydrate pit." When my office staff did a hair analysis on Sue we found her to be deficient in both chromium and vanadium, two minerals essential for proper blood sugar metabolism. After undergoing corrective nutritional therapy and implementing my *Eat, Drink and Be Healthy* program the blood sugar swings were under control and in the process she lost weight and the terrible moods swings stopped.

The same is true with so many children in this country diagnosed with ADD and ADHD. The primary problem (though this condition can have many contributing factors) I have seen with the majority of children so diagnosed who have come into my office is hypoglycemia and allergies to red dye and blue dye. The standard medical procedure for ADD rarely involves checking the child's blood sugar (via a glucose tolerance test) but simply prescribing the class II drug Ritalin to mask the symptoms.

Remember Ritalin does not cure ADD. It only covers up the symptoms. It is kind of like taking aspirin for a headache. You don't have a deficiency of aspirin, but you take it to mask the symptoms. By the way, Ritalin is such a strong drug it is in the same class as morphine. How many caring parents would allow a physician to routinely prescribe morphine to their child?

If you want to know more about this topic call my office and order my *Eat, Drink and Be Healthy* program. It contains 8 audio tapes on health, my wife's cookbook, and cutting-edge reports I have written on natural therapies for high blood pressure, diabetes, cancer, depression, ADD, and prostrate impotency and infertility in men. This nutritionally-based program has worked for thousands and it can work for you also.

It is difficult for me not to give you as much information as I possibly can concerning your health needs, but for now let's get back to glucagon.

Glucagon is secreted by the pancreas to raise blood glucose levels by freeing stored glucose from the muscle tissues and the liver. It also stimulates the breakdown of fat and eventually puts a halt to fat storage.

The Formula to Put into Place

Now here's the formula we must put into place in our body chemistry:

Increase levels of glucagon

and

Decrease levels of insulin

How can this be accomplished? Two things must occur simultaneously:

1. You must reduce your high-glycemic-index carbohydrates and increase the percentage of low-fat protein at mealtimes.

(High-glycemic-index carbs are those that turn to sugar quickly—we'll have more on that in a few paragraphs.)

2. You must exercise regularly.

Reduced carbohydrate meals reduce the production of insulin, allowing the protein that is consumed to stimulate glucagon production. By the way, exercise stimulates glucagon production perhaps even better than a low-carb meal.

The scientists in the 1980s were right when they told us the body was designed to get its fuel primarily from carbohydrates. They simply went too far when they advised us to overdose on them. They were also right to warn us about the dangers of a high-fat diet, but they were wrong to put a curse on *all* fats (which includes essential fatty acids).

Not All Carbohydrates are High-Glycemic-Index

You may be asking, "What are high-glycemic-index carbohydrates?"

Not all carbohydrates produce extreme insulin reactions. Researchers have carefully classified various foods according to the amount of blood sugar they produce in the bloodstream over a three-hour period. Some carbohydrates produce a high-insulin output—they are called high-glycemic foods. Other carbohydrates, called low-glycemic foods, generate very little insulin in the bloodstream. These low-glycemic foods may be eaten at will, in virtually any quantity desired. They include most fresh vegetables and some fruits.[5]

At the mean, or center, of the Glycemic Index are flour and wheat products such as whole wheat and white bread, which have an index of 100. Any food with a Glycemic Index of 70 and above is considered a high-glycemic index food, an insulin promoter, and a glucagon inhibitor. Foods such as processed grains, bread, most pastas, biscuits, pancakes, cereals, cakes, white rice, and refined flour are high-glycemic. They should be considered luxuries and *never* eaten if you are trying to lose fat. They certainly cannot be the mainstay of a diet that is aimed at maintaining maximum fat loss!

What is the very practical conclusion to the best dietary intake for maximum fat-loss?

1. Eat lots of fresh vegetables and fresh fruits (low-glycemic).

2. Continue to eat moderate amounts of lean proteins.

This eating regimen must be coupled with diligent exercise, sufficient amounts of pure water, and vitamin and mineral supplements.

Keeping Your Muscles Healthy While Reducing Carb Intake

One of the best ways to avoid small, flat, or flabby muscles as you lose fat is to eat your healthy meals *after* exercise times. This is also the best time to take certain supplements discussed in a later chapter.

For up to two hours after intense exercise, the body works to restore glycogen directly to the muscles, bypassing the liver and other storage sites, including fat cells. At the same time, you need to make sure that you rehydrate your muscle cells by drinking sufficient pure water.[6]

SIX HEALTHY MEALS—A BASIC KEY

Let's return to the basic key related to your calorie intake. Divide your calories across six healthy meals a day. Space those meals evenly. And eat the right things at each meal.

Even if you don't understand all the biochemistry and physiology at work, you *can* know what to do to put into place the right chemical process!

Precisely how *much* protein you should eat is the subject of the next chapter.

KEY #4:

Eat sufficient high-quality protein at every meal.

6

YOU REALLY *ARE*
WHAT YOU EAT

nlike tobacco, alcohol, and illegal drugs—which a person can quit cold turkey and never take again—food is required for basic survival. A person must eat.

It's up to you to decide what you will eat, and in what proportion. The overriding principle to follow is this: Every meal should have both protein, carbohydrates, and fat.

In this chapter we'll deal with your protein intake.

GETTING ALL THE PROTEIN YOUR BODY NEEDS

You need to consume one gram of protein per pound of *lean body mass* per day in order to provide the body with the amino acid building blocks necessary to support muscle growth.

Note that lean body mass is not your total weight—it's the percentage of your weight that is not fat. To determine your lean body mass, you need to calculate your BMI (which gives you the approximate percentage of your body that is fat). Multiply your BMI by your weight and you'll have the actual number of pounds of your body weight that should be considered fat. Subtract this from your total body weight and you will have your lean body mass. (Water is fairly evenly distributed throughout the body in all vessels, cells, and tissues so it is not a factor in these calculations. You can also use your body fat caliper to determine lean muscle mass.)

As an example: A man who has 150 pounds of lean body mass needs 150 grams of protein a day. The target calorie level for such a man would be about 600 calories a day of protein. The remainder of the diet would be about 800 calories from carbohydrates and 600 calories of fat for a total of 2,000 calories. If you break this down over six healthy meals, you'll find about 30 grams or 100 calories of protein at each meal.

When to Eat Protein.

The two most important times to eat protein are right before bed and when you get up. The protein you eat in the evening decreases the muscle-wasting effects that your body experiences overnight. If you are eating only about two hundred calories at night, make sure that they are nearly all lean protein, with only a few calories devoted to carbohydrates.

Exercise Maximizes the Benefits of Protein.

When you are losing fat, you need even more protein because your body burns more protein on a low-calorie diet.[1]

Aim at one gram of protein per pound of body weight each day while you are engaged in a rigorous exercise program to augment your fat-loss program. You must be exercising regularly in order for this protein to do its maximum work in your body. If you aren't exercising, this amount of protein will be counter-productive.

START YOUR DAY WITH A PROTEIN SHAKE

Protein powders have been around for decades, and have been increasingly popular among those who are health-conscious for at least forty years. The good news about these powders is that new protein technologies are increasing both their effectiveness and taste.

The rule of thumb for protein powders is this: The higher the protein quality, the easier it is for the body to use the amino acids. It is very important that you get high-quality protein into your body. Today's protein powders often have a high-quality profile, which means they supply adequate percentages of all twenty amino acids.

Here is an overview of the basic products available:

Whey Protein

It is important to note that if it is an animal-based protein it may contain antibiotics or steroids. Be sure to find out before you buy a particular brand. Also, a lot of protein powders contain the artificial sweetener Nutrasweet or aspartame. These should never be used. I'll discuss more about artificial sweeteners later.

Whey is found in milk and was originally isolated as a by-product of cheese production. It is loaded with protein, dissolves well in water, is highly digestible, and has a better amino acid profile than even the highly regarded egg-white protein. New technologies have allowed for whey protein to be converted to powder form without undesirable lactose, fat, and cholesterol components of naturally occurring whey. Make sure in choosing a whey protein powder that a low-heat, micro-filtration, or ion exchange process was used in its manufacturing. (You'll find this information on the label or as part of the packaging.)

Whey protein has immunoglobulin proteins that supplement the body's immune system. It has the highest concentration of branched-chain amino acids of any single protein source, it enhances the production of glutathione in the body (a powerful antioxidant), and it has excellent solubility and digestibility.

The two main negatives to whey protein are that it can be several times more expensive than some other protein sources, and that it can come from a dairy source that may contain bovine growth hormone or antibiotics, both of which should be avoided.[2]

Soy Protein

Soy has never been big among those who take nutrition or bodybuilding seriously. For years it was considered an inferior form of protein, but recent technologies have greatly improved the digestibility and effectiveness of this type of protein. The soy-based protein powders tend to have a concentration of the top five amino acids. Soy protein may also help reduce nitrogen loss and enhance fat loss during low-calorie dieting. Male lab animals have experienced greater testosterone and growth-hormone excretion as well as muscle growth. Female lab animals, on the other hand, have actually lost weight and showed a decrease in testosterone and growth hormone. A number of studies have shown that soy has cholesterol-lowering and triglyceride-lowering effects. Soy-protein also seems to make the blood a little thinner, which may help support circulation and nutrient delivery of glucose to muscles.[3]

Soy protein seems to give the thyroid hormones a boost and it has been shown to have anticancer properties. Soy protein is what my family and I use most of the time.

Egg Protein

Egg protein powders were considered the highest quality proteins available for more than thirty years. Even though these powders seem to have been replaced in popularity by the whey-and newly improved soy powders, you should still find comfort that egg protein has the best "cookability" factor of the three! You can't cook whey, casein, or soy powder in the microwave or in a Teflon-coated pan. You *can* cook egg whites!

Of all the whole-food proteins available, egg whites are at the top of the list. They have higher quality protein than skim milk, cottage cheese, and chicken breast meat! Egg-white protein has an outstanding amino acid profile. Furthermore, the egg-white powder products mix easily, cook in the microwave in seconds, and taste good. A few manufacturers of egg-white products have even added L-glutamine. Look for it on the label. (These products are not only good for direct consumption, but they work very well in baking.) As with whey, egg protein may come from chickens that have had hormones or antibiotics injected into them or their feed. Be cautious.

Casein

Casein is the "other" milk protein (besides whey). Cottage cheese is really nothing more than fresh, unadulterated casein with a bit of calcium and lactose along for the ride. Nonfat cottage cheese is the best source of quality casein protein available anywhere. Its slow travel time through the digestive tract yields good absorption of amino acids and it has a high glutamine content (higher than whey, soy, and egg proteins). Casein has also been shown to increase neurotransmitter activity in the brain. It can help with the absorption of threonine, glutamine, and arginine, which are helpful to muscle cells. I only recommend organic cottage cheese.

And One to Avoid for Right now.

There's a new protein source that is hitting the market: wheat-protein hydrolysate. It is very high in natural glutamine and is soluble in cold water, easily digestible, and has a good amino acid profile. The stuff tastes horrible, however. Trust me, you will be disappointed. The manufacturers may eventually do something about the taste of this stuff, which is why I'm mentioning it at all.

Combine Protein Sources.

Rather than concentrate on using just one type of protein powder in making a protein shake, you may mix your proteins while you are in a fat-loss program. You may want to mix them in each drink, or alternate them among days. I recommend this blend in equal proportions (one third each):

- Soy-protein

- Whey protein

- Casein protein

Save your egg-white proteins for times when you actually want something to chew rather than drink.

This combination produces a strong cluster effect of amino acids to support muscle metabolism and growth. It has a good antioxidant effect and is actually higher in biological value than any one of the individual protein sources alone. The combination especially seems to boost the immune system.

Mix Your Protein Shakes with Fruits.

A protein-drink smoothie can be made by mixing your protein drink with frozen strawberries or frozen chunks of banana. You can also make a good protein shake by using fresh fruit and ice cubes.

You might also try mixing your protein powders in vegetable juices of various kinds (especially homemade juices such as carrot juice and celery juice). Vegetable juice gives an entirely new flavor to the idea of protein.

Give It a Try.

Some people seem reluctant to make protein shakes because they are concerned about getting too much protein, which may lead to kidney problems.

The job of the kidneys is to excrete urea, which is formed from ammonia, which in turn comes from the protein in our diet. The kidneys, however, were *designed* to do just this work. The key to assisting general kidney health is to drink sufficient water. A continual flushing of all toxins from the body is necessary, especially during fat loss. Keep up your water intake and you should have no kidney problems related to your protein consumption.

What about osteoporosis and protein? Osteoporosis seems to be related to many risk factors and there are no studies that show a clear link between a *moderate*-protein diet and this degeneration of bone tissue. It is extremely unlikely that you will consume more protein than your body can use if you stay within the calorie range recommended in this book and divide your protein intake over six meals a day.

Please be careful with the strictly *high*-protein diets. They can be very detrimental and can impact liver and kidney function as well as cause osteoporosis. *Moderate* protein consumption, however, has not been shown by any medical or scientific study to have negative effects—it is moderate protein consumption that I am advocating in a maximum fat-loss program. I do not recommend a ketogenic or high protein Atkins type of diet. I consider this program to be a disaster waiting to happen to your body chemistry and digestive system.

WHOLE-FOOD SOURCES OF PROTEIN

There are many good sources for protein beyond protein powders, of course. Following is a quick survey of the most popular protein foods. Please make certain that when you are purchasing whole-food proteins that you buy free-range or organic products that are free of all animal-growth hormones and antibiotics.

Chicken

The proverbial chicken breast is still the number one choice of nonpowder protein. Chicken breast meat is low in fat and high in amino acids. Take off the skin and grill the meat.

Turkey

Turkey is highly nutritious and lean. Watch out for ground turkey, however. Make sure you are getting ground turkey *breast*, not ground turkey with skin or dark meat. Ground turkey breast has only

1 to 2 percent fat, but turkey with skin or dark meat may have as much as 20 percent fat. (That's about equal to ice cream!)

Fish

The fat content of fish various greatly, depending not only on the species of fish but whether they've been packed in oil or water. The fish to avoid are herring, mackerel, pompano, sardines, and shad—which can have more than 10 grams of fat per serving! Also high in fat are catfish, shark, and bluefish, which have between 5 and 10 grams of fat per serving. Don't eat these species.

Feel free to indulge in lean fish such as cod, haddock, orange roughy, perch, pike, red snapper, rockfish, and sea bass. If you are eating canned fish, look for water-packed fish and rinse the fish to eliminate as much sodium and fat as possible.

My wife's cookbook contains a complete list of fish, meat, and poultry that are safe to eat and those that should be avoided.

Eggs

When choosing to eat egg products, I believe you are wisest to stick with egg *whites*. Whole eggs do have a high amount of lecithin, which emulsifies the cholesterol in egg yolks, but nonetheless, the real protein power of eggs lies in the white of the egg.

Organ Meats

For the most part, stay away from them. Although liver may be high in iron, it is also very high in arachidonic acid (fat) and cholesterol. You're better off getting your iron from another source. A major function of the liver is to detoxify the body. Why would you want to eat an organ that is full of toxins?

Nuts

I suggest you avoid nuts as a snack. They are natural and can contain a lot of protein, but for the most part they are also very high in fat. The one exception is chestnuts, which have only about 8 percent fat.

Many people seem to have read that walnuts are low in fat. Actually, the study that led to this conclusion was a study that compared walnuts to beef and butter. Yes, walnuts *are* lower in fat than beef and butter, but they still are high in fat and should be eaten sparingly.

Milk

Organic nonfat milk and fat-free milk products are fine. Anything else should be avoided, even 2 percent, reduced-fat, and other low-fat milks. The only exception is for children under the age of two. They need to be on high-fat milk daily to ensure proper brain, nerve, and mylein formation. However, I prefer raw certified goat's milk for children and adults. It greatly reduces allergies and has not been linked to juvenile diabetes.

I have been amazed at the number of people who think that by turning to frozen yogurt they are avoiding the fat of ice cream. Some varieties of frozen yogurt have as many as 8 grams of fat per cup! Then, too, there's virtually no way you can tell the fat content of the local neighborhood yogurt stand's product. If the frozen yogurt is 1 gram of fat or less per serving, you may want to treat yourself occasionally. Don't make it a habit, however, and make sure you know with certainty that the frozen yogurt you are being served has one or fewer grams of fat per serving.

Don't use frozen yogurt or any product sweetened with aspartame or any artificial sweetener. If you ask at the counter and they don't know the ingredients, don't buy it. By the way, most frozen yogurt is loaded with sugar.

Organic Beef

Many books about weight loss recommend that a person eliminate beef from the diet, or cut way back on beef. I'd like to say a word in favor of beef.

Today's beef products are much lower in fat, calories, and cholesterol than products before 1980. One study showed that the average beef product today is 27 percent lower in fat than it was in 1986. Beef is a great source of protein, B-vitamins, creatine, zinc, and iron. Lean beef is about 72 percent water, 20 percent protein, and only about 7 percent fat.

Lean beef is very close to a chicken breast or fish (flounder) in cholesterol for a three-ounce serving. Check out the numbers below for a nutrient comparison:

	Total Fat	Saturated Fat	Cholesterol
Chicken Breast	3.0 grams	0.9 grams	72 mg
Top Round Steak	4.0 grams	1.0 gram	71 mg
Turkey (light/dark)	5.0 grams	1.6 grams	64 mg
Top Sirloin	6.1 grams	2.4 grams	76 mg
Chicken Thigh	9.3 grams	2.6 grams	81 mg

Beef is highly digestible—it is 97 percent digestible compared to 89 percent for flour and 65 percent for most vegetables. Digestibility refers to the proportion of food that becomes available to the body as absorbed nutrients. Beef and other protein foods remain in the stomach longer than fruits and vegetables and give people a feeling of fullness for a longer period of time.

Fat content varies according to various cuts of beef. Take a look at these simple comparisons for a three-ounce portion:

	Calories	Protein Grams	Fat Grams
Brisket	189	27	8
Flank Steak	213	23	9
Lean Ground (10% fat)	169	22	9
T-Bone Steak	182	24	9
Top Sirloin Steak	165	26	6
Rib Eye Steak	191	24	10

Eye Round	143	25	4
Round Tip	157	24	6
Top Round	153	27	4
Shank (crosscuts)	171	29	5

Be sure to trim away all excess fat from your meat before cooking it. A butcher can do this for you. Then trim again before you *eat* your meat.

Cook your beef using a light coating of olive oil spray in the pan so you don't add any extra oils or fat to the process. Most beef is best grilled or seared, using a very high temperature to brown the outer layer of the meat to seal in the juices. After searing, turn the heat down to medium and cook until the desired doneness. If you are using a roasting pan, be sure to use an insert rack so the grease drains away from the meat and the meat is not steeped in its own fat.

Always drain away any grease before adding cooked beef (such as ground beef or beef pieces) to stews or sauces. Kosher beef is the best to buy.

AIDS TO HELP PROTEIN DIGESTION

The digestion and absorption process for whole proteins is really quite remarkable. More than 90 percent of the proteins we take into our bodies are eventually broken down into amino acids and protein peptides and absorbed through the intestine for building body cells and providing energy. The digestion of proteins is a complicated process, however, and it takes time and relatively large amounts of energy to complete.

The higher the percentage of protein intake in the form of protein peptides, the greater the digestion, absorption, and bioavailability of the amino acids. There are new products that help to jump-start the digestion process of whole proteins by creating peptides. They also release a large number of branched-chain free-form amino acids into the intestine, allowing them to be absorbed more quickly. This is a product that can be added to powdered protein drinks to make them even more effective.[4]

CALCULATING PROTEIN GRAMS

Many calorie and gram counters are available on the market. (One is provided in the *Maximum Fat Loss Workbook*.) Take a look at what you intend to eat for protein at each meal and do some math. Add up the protein grams for each meal and make sure that you haven't exceeded the total in grams of your lean muscle mass.

Don't just guess at this. Get out your calculator.

Again, your first meal of the day and your last meal should be high in protein (but not all protein).

These protein grams are to be balanced with carbohydrate grams, our next order of business.

KEY #5:

Eat low-glycemic-index carbohydrates at every meal.

7

GET THERMODYNAMICS
ON YOUR SIDE

Thermodynamics is the term used to describe the calories that are expended by the body as it digests food. Thermogenesis results in the burning of more calories.

The good news for most people is that digestion by itself requires calories. The more often the body must break down food, the more efficient the body's thermodynamic response system becomes.[1]

Here's an example: If you eat one hundred calories of carbohydrates, your body uses about twenty-three calories just to process that food. Your body uses even more calories to process protein, but only three calories to process fat. Low-glycemic index foods may actually require more calories to process them than they contain. This is one time when negative numbers are really great assets!

SOME FOODS ARE FAT-BURNERS

Another way of saying this is that some foods are fat-burners. They can actually help you lose weight by stoking the internal fires of your body's metabolism. These foods boost your body's natural fat-burning ability. And remember, it's always fat we want to burn up, not our muscles.

These are among the vegetables that are excellent fat-burners:

- alfalfa sprouts
- artichoke
- asparagus
- bamboo shoots
- bean sprouts
- bok choy
- broccoli
- Brussels sprouts
- cabbage
- cauliflower
- celery
- chard
- cucumbers
- eggplant
- greens (such as beet, collard, dandelion, mustard, turnip
- lettuce
- okra
- parsley
- pea pods
- peppers (green, red, chiles)
- pickles (dill)
- radishes
- sauerkraut
- soy beans
- spinach
- string beans
- summer squash
- tomatoes
- zucchini

Please note that arthritis sufferers need to avoid eggplant, tomatoes, potatoes, and bell peppers. These items often inflame the joints of some arthritis patients.

These are also good vegetables to include in your eating plan, although less often:

- beans
- beets
- carrots
- corn
- onions
- peas
- pumpkin
- yellow turnip
- winter squash
- yams

When it comes to vegetables, think green and yellow. Vegetables of these colors, overall, have about a fourth of the calories of more starchy vegetables.

Certain vegetables also have other very helpful health benefits to the fat-loss process. For example, cabbage, cauliflower, broccoli, Brussels sprouts, green leafy vegetables, beans, and other legumes have been shown to have beneficial effects in lowering insulin secretion after a meal.

Perhaps not surprisingly, hot red pepper (capsaicin) is considered a thermogenic food, helping the body to burn more calories. Try it, judiciously, in place of salt. Cayenne pepper and dried red pepper flakes are convenient sources of capsaicin.

Fat-Burner Research

Several supplements are mentioned in a later chapter to help with fat-burning. These may be very helpful to you in burning off body fat.

Of special interest to fat-loss experts are studies involving beta-3 site receptors. These receptors are found in a type of human fat called brown fat. The theory is that if these receptors can be kicked into high gear, a great deal of fat can be burned from the body. Watch for developments in both thermogenetics and beta-3 site receptors research. By the way, if you want to be on my mailing list for future updates, call my office for details.

FRUIT AS A SOURCE OF CARBOHYDRATES

Fruits are a good carbohydrate source—in moderation. Every person should have a couple of servings of fruit a day. My favorite choice is to have one to two pieces of fruit during the day and to mix one portion of fruit in my morning protein drinks.

Fructose is the simple sugar found in fruit. Your should be aware that while fructose has a low glycemic index and a low insulin response in comparison to sucrose, an excessive consumption of fructose may be counterproductive. A high-fructose diet may lead to insulin resistance and lower the benefit the body receives from antioxidants. Eat fruit, but stay primarily with the low glycemic fruit.

Good fruit choices include the following:

- 3 medium fresh apricots
- 1 apple
- 1 banana
- 1/2 cup blackberries
- 1/2 cup blueberries
- 1 cup boysenberries
- 1 cup cranberries
- 2 figs
- 1/2 grapefruit
- 2 kiwifruit
- 2 lemons or limes
- 1/2 mango
- 1/2 melon: cantaloupe
- 1/4 melon: casaba, crenshaw, honeydew
- 1 nectarine
- 1 orange
- 1 cup papaya
- 1 peach
- 1 pear
- 1/4 fresh pineapple
- 2 plums
- 1/2 cup raspberries
- 1 cup strawberries
- 2 tangerines
- 1 cup watermelon

Fruit Juice

I do not recommend that *any* juice be a part of your eating plan while you are trying to lose body fat. As part of a maintaince program, some juice is acceptable but it must be natural, unsweetened, and taken in small quantities. (The same goes for vegetable juices.) Think fresh, not canned. Even as part of a maintenance program avoid or greatly limit grape juice and prune juice, which are extremely high in sugar.

Dried Fruits

Dried fruits contain concentrated calories. Because they have less water content, pieces of dried fruit are also less filling. You would probably not be able to eat three whole apricots in the time it takes you to read this page of the book, but you could easily, and almost unconsciously, eat ten dried apricots in that time. The difference would be about 350 calories *more* in eating the dried apricots!

Keep your portion of dried fruit under two ounces. (Some dried fruits are treated with sulphur dioxide, which can aggravate asthma in some people—use caution if you are asthmatic.)

LIMIT GRAINS AND STARCHY VEGETABLES

As we mentioned earlier, when you want to prepare an animal for slaughter, you feed that animal highly processed carbohydrates—usually high-carb grain products. Sadly, most Americans are also eating a ready-for-slaughter diet.

It's time to cut out *all* potatoes, rice, pasta, and bread, and the products that use these foods.

In their place, choose brown rice and wild rice. These are acceptable carbohydrate sources if (1) these products are eaten in balance with protein, and (2) these items are not over eaten, which means they are not eaten too frequently or in too large a quantity.

Whole and parboiled rice have significantly lower insulin-stimulating effects than wheat. In fact, some research shows that high-amylose varieties of rice may be useful in lowering insulin secretion after a meal.[2]

When eating grains, consider using these items:

- oatmeal
- 2 Tbs. flaxseed
- whole-grain Kashi
- wild rice

When to Eat High Glycemic Fruits

If high-glycemic fruit is eaten it should be consumed one to two hours *after* a weight-training workout. At that time, the body is somewhat depleted of glycogen, and insulin sensitivity is up so the body can make the best use of those carbohydrates at that time to replenish muscle tissue. This is why I use bananas in my protein shake.

If you spike your insulin level when your body fuel stores are low—such as after a workout—the nutrients from your meal are driven mainly into muscle cells to replace energy stores there and to deliver the amino acids needed for recuperation and growth. However, if you spike your insulin levels when these muscle energy stores are full—which is most of the day—then a good portion of the carbs and protein are diverted to fat cells for storage.

The only time in a day when you should spike your insulin production is following your workout. If you must eat high-glycemic-index carbohydrates, you should eat them only *once* a day and, very specifically, thirty minutes to two hours after a workout. If you are exercising first thing in the morning, this means that your *breakfast* meal after your workout is the meal where you should include any high glycemic food.

The rest of your meals should be protein with low-glycemic-index carbohydrates (such as peas, kidney, or black beans, barley, and yogurt) and a little fat.

Do not eat any high glycemic products after six o'clock at night (even whole-wheat bread, pasta, or bagels). Your last meal of the day should have only low-glycemic-index carb foods—in other words, green and yellow vegetables.

CLUSTERS AND PERCENTAGES OF NUTRIENTS

The latest research in nutrition is aimed at the ways in which clusters of nutrients and foods work together to produce effects in the body. The newest studies involve the ratios of foods we consume (proteins, fats, and carbohydrates) for the maximum benefit.

Barry Sears, a noted researcher, believes we should consume 40 percent carbohydrates, 30 percent protein, and 30 percent fat. He doesn't really specify which types of proteins are preferred but he advocates that a person only choose carbohydrates that are fifty and below on a glycemic index. (Dr. Ann deWees Allen, another noted researcher in this area, believes the glycemic index cut-off point should be seventy and below.) I believe the cut-off point should be sixty and below.

My general recommendation to my clients is a daily consumption of between thirty-five and forty-five percent of their total diet in carbohydrates, with the vast majority (70% or more) of those being low-glycemic-index carbs. Remember, protein and carbohydrates have four calories per gram.

Fat should be kept between 25 and 35 percent of total calorie intake Remember, fat has nine calories per gram. But this amount is to include all supplemental fats used including olive oil for cooking and cod liver oil for providing essential fatty acids. I will discuss more about these fats later.

Protein needs to be one gram per pound of body weight. That should be equal to 30-40 percent of total calorie needs.

Once again, you need to do your math. Count your grams! As is true for protein grams, charts of carbohydrate grams are readily available on the market. (There's one in the *Maximum Fat Loss Workbook*.)

A good mix is around forty grams of carbohydrate to around thirty grams of protein—if you are eating the *best* of the lowest carbs.

There are some carbs that simply should *never* be eaten. We go there next.

A SAMPLING OF THE GLYCEMIC INDEX

You can find a complete Glycemic Index in the *Maximum Fat Loss Workbook*. Basically, any food that has a glycemic index of greater than one hundred is considered to be a rapid inducer of insulin. Foods between seventy and ninety-nine are moderate inducers of insulin. And foods between forty and sixty-nine are called reduced inducers of insulin. Those foods with a glycemic index below forty are ones that you can usually eat to your heart's desire because they may require more energy to digest than they contribute to the body. They have virtually no impact on insulin production.

Below I have listed several categories of carbohydrates and food products in each category that have a glycemic index of seventy or below:

BREAKFAST CEREALS
all-bran

rice bran

CEREAL GRAINS
barley

rice (instant, boiled 1 minute)

bulgur

wheat kernels

FRUITS AND FRUIT PRODUCTS
apple

orange

apple juice

peach, fresh

apricots

peach, canned in water

cherries

pear, fresh

grapefruit

pear, canned in water

grapefruit juice

pineapple juice

LEGUMES
baked beans, canned

lima beans, baby frozen

beans, dried, not specified

pinto beans

black-eyed peas

pinto beans, canned

butter beans (w/o sucrose)

soy beans

chick peas (garbanzo beans)

soy beans, canned

chick peas, canned

split peas, yellow boiled

navy beans

tomato

kidney beans

lentil, canned

lentils

VEGETABLES
cabbage

green onions

celery

hot peppers

peas, green

peas, dried

Chinese cabbage

radishes

cucumber

zucchini

SALAD GREENS
endive

romaine lettuce

lettuce

spinach

KEY #6:

Purge your life of the foods and beverages that are bad for you.

8

DUMP OUT THAT
SUGAR BOWL

We've been dealing primarily with what you should eat on a fat-loss program. There are a number of things you also should *not* eat. Sugar is one of those things that has devastating effects on fat loss.

A big double whammy occurs when simple sugars and heated fats are consumed together. This combination is routinely found in fried foods, candy, cookies, cakes, sweet rolls, donuts, and so forth. Not only does the person who consumes simple sugars and heated fat experience dramatic increases in blood fats, but also higher rates of fat storage and weight gain and a decreased metabolic rate.

In other words, a donut, and cup of coffee is *not* breakfast. It is an injection of ill health!

One nutrition physician has called sugar "slow suicide." I'm not sure it is going to remain all that slow as the years progress. The average American intake of added sugar—the white stuff, not naturally occurring sugars in fruits—is twenty and a half teaspoons a day. That adds up to sixty-eight and a half pounds of sugar a year. And that is considered to be a conservative estimate.

When the total sugar is calculated—added sugars as well as naturally occurring sugars—the amount becomes more than 152 pounds per year. Many people are literally eating their weight in sugar every year.[1]

Certainly one of the major reasons for this high consumption of sugar in the American diet is the proliferation of soft drinks in the last six decades. An average soda has the equivalent of ten teaspoons of sugar. Talk about a liquid candy bar! The average teenage boy drinks 3.5 twelve-ounce sodas in a day—one out of ten teenage boys drinks *seven* cans a day. That's thirty-five to seventy teaspoons of sugar! Girls in the same age group drink an average of 2.5 cans of sugared sodas a day. Overall, every American drinks more than fifty-four gallons of soda a year. Sodas, of course, are just one source of sugar. Add to that snack foods, candy bars, and fruit drinks and the amount of refined sugar our children and teens are consuming is staggering.

Furthermore, when people eat a lot of sugar, they tend to feel far less hungry for the things their bodies need most. Research has shown that those who consume the highest amounts of sugar take in the lowest amounts of vitamins A, C, B12, and folate, as well as calcium, phosphorus, magnesium, zinc, and iron. Deficiencies in these nutrients generally arise from the fact that those who eat high-sugar diets tend to eat fewer fruits, vegetables, and meats.[2]

A RISING EPIDEMIC OF DIABETES

Given our massive consumption of sugar, I am not at all surprised that diabetes is reaching epidemic proportions in our nation, even though many misinformed physicians continue to advocate that dietary sugar has no connection to behavior problems, mood swings, depression, or the increased incidence of adult-onset diabetes. In fact, the federal government says that the only health problem linked to sugar is tooth decay! The Sugar Association, with the support of the American Dietetic Association, holds a position that sugar is a healthy, low-calorie sweetener that is no different than any other carbohydrate, given it has only fifteen calories per tea-spoon.

I strongly disagree.

Diabetes falls into two types. Type I, which is often referred to as juvenile diabetes since it occurs early in life, involves a complete failure of the body to produce any insulin. Insulin injections are required to provide adequate levels of the hormone.

Type II diabetes is called adult-onset diabetes or non-insulin dependent diabetes. It is sometimes referred to as NIDDM: non-insulin-dependent diabetes mellitus. Type II is by far the most common form of diabetes—between 90 and 95 percent of all diabetics have Type II diabetes. It generally is diagnosed in adulthood since it takes a long time to develop in the body. In fact, research published in the United Kingdom estimates that those who develop Type II diabetes may have been suffering insulin resistance for as long as twelve years prior to actual diagnosis.

Type II diabetes begins with insulin resistance. Higher and higher amounts of insulin are required for the cells to open up and allow blood sugar in. For a while, the pancreas is usually able to produce the ever-increasing amounts of insulin required. Over time, however, the quality of the insulin produced decreases and eventually the pancreatic cells start to lose their ability to produce enough insulin. That's when Type II becomes easily diagnosed.

Adult-onset diabetes is also growing in epidemic proportions. There has been an increase of between 600 percent and 1,000 percent in just the last sixty years in our nation, and the disease is currently escalating at a phenomenal rate of six percent a year. That rate shows every sign of increasing in the years ahead.

Type II diabetes was practically unheard of in young people until just the last few years, but it is also now growing at an alarming rate. The long-term damage that elevated blood sugar levels have on blood vessels throughout the body is showing up even in thirty-year-olds: heart attacks, strokes, blindness, and amputations. One study done in

San Antonio showed an increase of nearly 6 percent in just one decade, with an increase of nearly 16 percent among the Mexican-American population.[3]

Diabetes Is a Killer.

Since medications are available for treating Type II diabetes, some people I've met don't seem too concerned about this disease. The truth is that diabetes is a very serious disease, with very serious consequences. It is the fourth leading cause of death in our nation.

The roller-coaster effects of constantly fluctuating blood sugar levels that I discussed earlier contribute to an increase in blood fat, high blood pressure, increased stickiness of the blood and clot formation, heart failure, polycystic ovary disease, nerve pain and degeneration, and damage to the small blood vessels (especially those in the eyes, kidneys, and lower limbs).

These results lead to very serious effects. Diabetes

- is the leading cause of blindness in people age twenty to seventy-four.
- is the leading cause of kidney failure.
- is responsible for as much as 60 percent of the impotency in males over age fifty.
- is responsible for severe nerve damage in up to 70 percent of all people with diabetes.
- is the major cause of stroke in the United States.
- is the leading cause of amputation of lower limbs.
- is known to increase the risk of heart disease by two to four times.

The best time to manage the disease, of course, is to do everything you can to prevent it. Elimination of excess body fat is one of the most important things you can do! If you want more information about natural treatment options for diabetes call my office and order a copy of the *Eat, Drink and Be Healthy* program.

Hypoglycemia Is Often a Forerunner.

There are those who say to me, "I have hypoglycemia, but at least I'm not diabetic." A very high percentage of hypoglycemics become diabetics. Deal with your hypoglycemia!

How do you know if you have or are developing a blood sugar problem?

Answer these questions:

- Do you awaken in the morning feeling irritable or a little depressed?

- Do you feel exhausted by emotional stress and strain?

- Do you feel nervous or jittery if a meal is late?

- Does your family consider you to be an emotional yo-yo? (In other words, do your moods change rapidly?)

- Does eating sweets seem to relieve these symptoms of exhaustion and nervousness?

- Do you sometimes feel as if you just can't think straight until you have something to eat?

If you answer yes to two or more of these questions, and especially to questions three and five, have your physician run a test to see if you are hypoglycemic or diabetic.

FAT LOSS AND SYNDROME X

Now for the exotic stuff. Exotic-sounding, that is. This is basic science and it's the reason you need to dump out that sugar bowl.

Insulin is secreted in two phases. A surge of insulin is initially released immediately following a meal, or when sugar or sweetness is detected in the mouth and digestive system. A second round of insulin is released shortly after a meal and continues to be released gradually for several hours.

Insulin opens up cell walls so blood sugar can enter them. For insulin to work properly, two things must happen. Insulin must be present in sufficient quantity and the cells in the body must remain responsive to its effects. When cells become unresponsive or resistant to the effects of insulin, *more* insulin is required. Insulin resistance is often related to obesity in a way that researchers are increasingly calling Syndrome X.

In Syndrome X, excess abdominal fat and fat that accumulates around the liver increase the amount of free fatty acids in the blood. As these fatty acids break down, they increase toxicity levels and that, in turn, causes two things: They inhibit the production of insulin, and they make muscle cells less sensitive to the available insulin.

Don't Dismiss This as Just Another Syndrome!

We seem to have a syndrome for just about everything in our society today. Syndrome X, however, is one that you need to take seriously, and it's one that you need to understand if you are going to be successful in a sustained fat-loss program.

Syndrome X is the name that scientists have given to a cluster of symptoms associated with the way insulin works with glucose in the bloodstream.

When excessive insulin is secreted—as in when we spike insulin secretion from overeating—the cells of our body can develop a resistance to insulin. When that happens, glucose is no longer adequately transported across cell membranes and the overall feeding of the body is impaired at the cellular level.

Syndrome X seems to affect as many as 25 percent of all adults who are not diabetic. That means about sixteen million adults in the

United States may have this condition. About one in five people who are insulin resistant seem to go on to become diabetic.

Diabetes isn't the only negative outcome. As many as half of those with Syndrome X may have problems with high blood pressure. Excessive insulin secretion can also lead to elevated triglyceride levels and lower HDL (good cholesterol) levels, both of which are major factors in coronary heart disease. Insulin resistance has been linked to some forms of cancer and also to the promotion of tumor growth. It also has been linked to colitis and Crohn's disease, both of which are inflammatory bowel disorders.

Who Is at Risk for Syndrome X?

Here are the top five factors related to the development of this syndrome:

1. A family history of Type II (adult-onset) diabetes
2. Apple-shaped obesity (most of a person's excess weight carried in the stomach and abdominal area). People with a high degree of insulin resistance typically demonstrate an increase in fat around the midsection of their bodies. If you are carrying most of your weight in your stomach area, you may be developing insulin resistance.
3. A diet high in saturated fat and simple carbohydrates
4. A sedentary lifestyle
5. Micronutrient imbalances

You may not be able to do much about the first factor, but you certainly can take charge of the other four factors!

The Benefits of Syndrome X Diagnosis

One of the major benefits in identifying Syndrome X is that physicians, and especially those physicians who are concerned about nutritional factors as they relate to disease and aging, now have an overall way of looking at a cluster of health problems. For example, physicians have known for years that what they recommend for lowering blood pressure may not, in and of itself, have much impact on lowering a person's risk for coronary heart disease. However, when a patient is put on a plan to lower the factors associated with Syndrome X, not only are patients with blood pressure problems helped, but the patients' coronary heart disease problems are also are helped!

A number of physical-exam and laboratory tests are used by physicians to diagnose Syndrome X, in addition to the five factors previously mentioned. Since nutritional imbalances are one of the factors, several tests that measure the presence of certain nutrients may be ordered by your physician if he suspects you have Syndrome X.

Help for Those with Syndrome X

There's good news in this story. Solely by losing weight, a person can often overcome insulin resistance. By eliminating all sucrose from the diet, a person can also often overcome insulin resistance and reverse the symptoms of Type II diabetes. This isn't true for everybody, but it's true for many people!

The nutrients that we currently know to be helpful in preventing and resolving Syndrome X include the following:

- Eicosapentaenoic acid (EPA) and docosapen-taenoic acid (DHA increase cell membrane responsiveness to insulin.

- Magnesium can have a significant effect on cell membrane responsiveness.

- Natural vitamin E seems to have a relationship to cell membrane responsiveness, and certainly has heart-protective qualities.

- Fiber has a significant effect on glycemic response.

- Chromium has a significant relationship to glucose disposal.

- Vanadyl sulfate helps in glucose transport.

Increased frequency of meals has been shown to improve insulin management and to lower both fat and insulin levels in the bloodstream. This is one of the main reasons I recommend six meals a day rather than two or three larger meals. You might also be interested in knowing that most professional body-builders are keenly aware of the relationship between muscle and blood sugar. They often eat six meals a day, restrict or eliminate all refined carbs (sugar), and eat foods higher in protein and complex carbohydrates in small amounts. All of these measures minimize their need for insulin, lower their body fat, and keep muscle mass in place.

Diets that are high in carbohydrates increase plasma triglyceride levels, cholesterol, and glucose concentrations. That's the underlying reason I recommend a diet that has reduced carbohydrates (and is based mainly on low-glycemic-index carbs) and an adequate amount of protein. Protein seems to blunt the rise of glucose in the bloodstream, causing less insulin to be secreted.

One of the key factors in Syndrome X is an increased risk of free radical damage. The antioxidants vitamin C, vitamin E, zinc, vitamin A, and selenium seem especially important in reversing these negative free radical effects.[4]

DUMP OUT YOUR SUGAR BOWL TODAY

Ready for a step of immediate action? Go immediately to your pantry and kitchen shelves and get rid of every bit of sugar you find—white or brown, granular, cube, or powdered.

Look for sucrose on every label. Eliminate all food products that are high in sucrose.

Plain and simple: You don't need *any* refined sugar in your diet. You are going to be far healthier without it and your fat-loss program is going to progress much faster and more smoothly if you simply get rid of this "white poison."

Slow suicide or fast change? The best response any person can make to elevated blood sugar levels is *fast change!* Don't delay in this. Dump out that sugar bowl and refuse to fill it again.

9

FIVE FOODS TO AVOID THE REST OF YOUR LIFE

My parents immigrated from Germany in 1952. My first language was German and I was raised on sauerkraut, Wiener schnitzel, and pork chops, plus mountains of hot dogs, sausage, and everything else ingenious Germans can make with pork and pork by-products.

I know my parents meant well, but they didn't know this diet was harmful to my health. The result, however, was devastating to me. At age twenty-seven, fresh out of graduate school at Florida State University, I nearly died of a heart condition, even though I was a highly conditioned athlete at the time.

How do I know my condition was caused, at least in part, by the pork products and high-fat luncheon meats I had consumed for years? Because when I stopped eating pork and processed meats (as well as shellfish), my life-threatening problems quickly improved and ultimately disappeared—even though my physicians could not touch the condition with conventional antibiotics and other drug therapies.

Pork is my number one choice of foods to eliminate from your diet in order not only to achieve maximum fat loss but to improve your overall health. The phrase "as fat as a pig" means just what it says.

ELIMINATE ALL PORK PRODUCTS

As far as I am concerned, diet problems don't get any worse than pork. In fact, if I could only tell you one food to change in your diet it would be this: Eliminate all pork products. The pig is unfit for human consumption! My opinion is that pigs were put here by God as scavenger feeders to help clean up the environment, but they were not put here to be eaten.

I am not the only scientist who holds this opinion. German professor Hans-Heinrich Reckeweg, M.D. published an article titled "The Adverse Influence of Pork Consumption on Health" and concluded very simply, "Pork should be regarded as an important homotoxin (human poison)."[1] You can't get much plainer than that!

One of the key problems with pork and high-fat luncheon meat is that these foods digest too quickly in the human digestive system. They are literally too "hot" for the body to handle. They slow down the body's ability to fight off diseases, including cancer, by impairing the immune system.

Over the years, I have found it interesting to discover just how many people do not think of pepperoni, the most frequently ordered pizza topping in America and formerly my first choice as well, as a pork product. Many processed meats, such as bologna and wieners and ham loaf, are pork. Check the labels of the foods you buy and avoid pork.

Perhaps the most famous of all pork products gives a double whammy. I'm talking about bacon. Not only is it pork, but the average bacon product is loaded with sodium nitrite. I am a biochemist and I know what happens to sodium nitrite when it reacts with stomach acids. Believe me, it is not a pretty picture. Sodium nitrite forms nitrosamines in the stomach—one of the most potent cancer-causing agents known to man. In my professional opinion, many cases of colon, pancreatic, and stomach cancer are directly related to the high-fat foods we eat—many of which are preserved with sodium nitrite—and the lack of fiber in the typical American diet.

A second chemical is also used frequently in the processing of meats: polycyclic hydrocarbons. The association between cancer and this chemical along with nitrosamines is so strong that the National Academy of Sciences issued a warning in 1982.[2] Sadly, too few Americans have heeded it.

The physical and biochemical problems with pork should be sufficient reasons not to eat pork, but to make matters worse, we use cancer-causing chemicals to process the stuff!

Several years ago I met a young girl in the Orlando International Airport who was on her way home from the Mayo Clinic. She told me she had been undergoing cancer therapy there. I asked her, "What did the physicians tell you about what you should and shouldn't eat?" She shrugged and said, "They told me to eat anything I want to eat."

I then asked, "Well, what foods do you like to eat." She looked up at me with her beautiful eyes and said, "All I eat are Twinkies, Ding Dongs, some hot dogs and diet sodas. That's it." I looked at this beautiful little girl wearing a ski cap to hide a head that was bald from chemotherapy and thought, *Why aren't our physicians reading the results of scientific research related to the foods we eat?* In many ways, because of how foods control hormones, and the chemical these foods contains, they *are* the drugs the vast majority of people take daily. And many of those drugs are ones that are counterproductive to health!

CUT OUT ALL SHELLFISH

Some of my favorite foods before my heart disease episode in my twenties were lobster, crab, shrimp, oysters, scallops, mussels, and-clams. I no longer consume any of the above.

There are two main reasons I have eliminated these foods from my life. First and foremost, I am inclined to exercise extreme caution any time God's Word warns about a particular food or food group, especially when there is so much evidence linking that food group to death rates. Second, I am specifically concerned when a food source may be contaminated by environmental factors.

In some cases, the probability of shellfish having toxemia or toxic problems may be low if the shellfish have been farm raised or harvested in clean waters. Unfortunately, however, most of the fish species and algae on which shellfish feed migrate freely from one part of the ocean to the other, picking up poisons and chemical contaminants along the way.[3]

Another factor to consider is that many species of shellfish are scavengers who roam the bottoms of ocean waters and feed on the carcasses of what has died in the ocean or lake. This is why the flesh of so many species of shellfish are found to be contaminated with mercury, lead, arsenic, carcinogens, and hundreds of synthetic and chemical contaminants. You don't have to be a biochemist to recognize that the toxins of these contaminants remain in the flesh of the shellfish and are passed upward in the food chain to those who eat the shellfish.

"But," you may argue, "if this is true, why aren't shellfish dying of cancer and other diseases?"

Actually, many shellfish species do suffer from major diseases and genetic abnormalities. Other shellfish, such as lobsters, are able to carry deadly carcinogens in their bodies and pass them along, while at the same time sequestering the carcinogens in their tissues in a way that prevents damage to their chromosomes.[4]

Another question to ask is: "How pure is the water these shellfish filter, and what is the environment for the phytoplankton they eat?" An oyster can filter up to fifty gallons of sea water in a day—and by "filter" I mean just that. It filters toxins *out* of the water—both chemical and bacteria—that are in the water, and those toxins remain in the oyster's flesh. We certainly know from studies involving land mammals, including humans, that watery vegetables and melons that are cultivated with highly contaminated water can cause sickness in mammals. Our vegetables are only as healthful as the water and soil that produce them. Polluted waters produce polluted creatures and vegetation.[5]

Shortly after I graduated from college I went with two friends to an exclusive country club for dinner. It was the club's "all-you-can-eat seafood buffet night" and we dove into the mounds of crab, lobster, shrimp, oysters, and numerous other items as if there were no tomorrow. There almost wasn't. For five full days I suffered from food poisoning. I have never been as violently nauseated and ill—and one of my friends suffered the same fate. I hate to think what we actually took into our bodies in the way of toxins.

One final warning: Not too long ago a scientific study was released about a bacteria named *Vibrio vulnificus.* It is in the same family of bacterium that causes cholera and it thrives in warm sea water. It is so virulent that it can infect people who expose an open wound to sea water containing the bacterium or to infected seafood, and it is particularly a danger for fish industry workers and food handlers.[6] When I say about shellfish that I don't touch the stuff, I mean this literally.

Please note that I am not saying that you should avoid eating *fish.* Fish and shellfish are two different classes of food. Certain fish are excellent choices for a low-fat, high-energy eating plan. Grouper, red snapper, orange roughy, and salmon are all fine food sources.

REMOVE ALL "JUNK FOOD" FROM YOUR GROCERY CART

I married a world-class junk-food eater. And I happily report that she is no longer consuming what she once did!

At the time I met my wife, Sharon, she was eating four to six candy bars a day. On our first date, she ordered *two* hot fudge desserts—the gooey kind with chocolate-fudge brownie covered with chocolate-fudge ice cream. Sharon, however, had never been informed about what was healthful and unhealthful to eat, and she was eager to learn to be healthy. She battled her way from chronic junk-food addiction to becoming an expert on healthy cooking and food choices. In fact, as I mentioned earlier, she has put together one of the best cookbooks on the market.[7]

You can't run a top-performance dragster on kerosene. For that matter, a genuine high-performance luxury car needs premium fuel. In the same way, your body is a finely tuned biochemical and bio-electrical creation designed by God for peak performance . . . but only if it is maintained properly.

Junk food is bad for you in two ways. First, these foods give you very little in the way of nutrients. When you fill your body with them, you tend not to eat the foods that truly are nutritional. Second, these foods can actually rob your system of vitamins, essential fats, minerals, and trace minerals.

Here are the telltale characteristics of a junk food:

A Long List of Preservatives on the Label

If you look at the label on a product and there is *anything* on that label that you cannot readily pronounce, don't buy the product. Nearly all junk foods are high in dangerous chemical preservatives.

One of my favorite stories to tell my audiences is the "Tale of the Fifteen-Year Old Twinkie." Several years ago I attended a health-food seminar sponsored by the National Health Federation and saw one display that had a lone Twinkie package on a shelf. I asked, "What's up with this Twinkie?" The man at the booth replied, "We're trying to determine its shelf life. No one knows for sure just what that is."

By now I was curious. "How long have you had it?" I asked.

I was shocked at his answer. "We've had it here at the seminar for the past fifteen years."

Just think about the implications of that statement—the Twinkie was so void of nutrients that even God's common single-celled bacteria couldn't find enough nutrients from it to sustain life.

Another one of the additives you should be especially concerned about is monosodium glutamate (MSG). This highly addictive flavor enhancer is often used in Chinese and other Far Eastern foods and has been associated with allergy problems and other health complications. Those who suffer an MSG allergic reaction can have breathing difficulties, chest pains, skipped heartbeats, and even partial paralysis. The glutamic acid component of MSG (monosodium glutamate) may also cause permanent brain damage. If you are planning on eating out at an Oriental restaurant, call ahead to see if they use MSG. Many Oriental restaurants have eliminated MSG but many more have not.[8]

Sugar as the First or Second Ingredient on the Label

For decades after sugar was first processed from cane, it bore a skull and crossbones danger sign and was considered to be a poison if consumed in large quantities. Virtually all junk foods are loaded with sugar, from soft drinks to candy bars.

The Use of Hydrogenated Fats

As a child, one of my favorite after-school snacks was a hefty portion of pork rinds and a soda, and followed by several peanut butter and jelly sandwiches chased with whole milk. Not only are pork rinds made of pork fat, but that pork fat had been *deep-fat-fried*. Talk about a double dose of trouble. Most chips and snack crackers, not to mention virtually all french fries and fried-chicken fast-food products are soaked with hydrogenated fats.

Do not be misled when reading a label—hydrogenated and *partially* hydrogenated fats are equally bad for you. (There's more on these fats a little later in this book.)

The problem with hydrogenated fats and fast-food restaurants is not only the fat itself, but the way it is used. The medical community has known for many years that once fat of any kind is heated to high temperatures for a period of time, it undergoes a chemical transformation and becomes carcinogenic (cancer causing).

The person who consumes the standard fast-food hamburger and fries is getting upwards of a thousand calories, virtually no vitamins or minerals, and woefully little protein. Rather, the person ends up with a stomach of calorie-laden foods that have no nutritional value and even has cancer-causing potential. No thanks.

The Use of Processed White Flour

You aren't going to find very many cake, cornbread, or cookie mixes without white flour. The same goes for many commercially packaged breads. It's really no wonder that breads often label themselves as "enriched" or "vitamins added" because the bleaching and leaching process of the flour used in manufacturing these breads virtually eliminates all nutrients and vitamins from the flour!

To get white bleached wheat flour, you have to strip totally the outer wheat kernel that contains all the nutrients and fiber—only the starchy middle section of the kernel remains. White flour paste used in kindergartens has about as much nutritional value.

Billions of dollars are spent in preparing and marketing foods for our grocery shelves that have extremely little to do with health and a great deal to do with money-making. The results are products that are not only *not* health-inducing but which actually may be proven to be health-destroying over time. Dr. Richard Brannon, chairman of the board of trustees of the International Academy of Preventive Medicine, has stated the situation well: "Most of the food in America today will support life, but it won't sustain health."

If you truly want to be *healthy* as you pursue maximum fat loss, you'll want to avoid junk foods. And, you'll want to keep junk foods out of the hands of your children.

AVOID HIGH-FAT DAIRY PRODUCTS

The fourth general food group to avoid in your quest for maximum fat loss is high-fat dairy products. Most Americans aren't aware of this fact: Whole milk is second only to beef as the largest source of saturated fat in the American diet.[9]

Of all the calories provided by whole milk, 50 percent are in the form of highly saturated milk fat. When it comes to cheese, 70 to 90 percent of the calories come from milk fat.

Most American adults have been taught from childhood: "Drink your milk." Many of us grew up believing that dairy products were one of the "four main food groups" and that the "milk group" was essential to a healthy life. We were taught that milk was "nature's most perfect food."

The fact is, we were victims of a very well-planned media blitz. While it is true that dairy products can be a source of calcium, the whole truth is that dairy foods are the most harmful of the traditional four food groups. They are not only high in fat and environmental contaminants, they are also deficient in fiber and carbohydrates.[10]

While we are mostly concerned about fat loss in this book, I would be negligent if I didn't also point out to you that after the age of about four years, most people naturally lose their ability to digest the carbohydrate known as lactose, which is found in milk. They no longer synthesize the digestive enzyme lactase that lines the small intestine, and the result is a lactose intolerance with symptoms of diarrhea, gas, and stomach cramps any time lactose-containing dairy products are consumed.

Many children, as well as adults, have strong allergies to cow's milk. Milk has been linked to allergic reactions that are respiratory in nature, with symptoms from nasal stuffiness and runny nose to asthmalike symptoms and inner ear inflammations. Others develop skin irritations such as hives, rashes, and more serious conditions. At least 50 percent of childhood iron-deficiency anemia and a significant number of cases of adult anemia has been linked to milk.[11]

If you really feel you must continue drinking milk, I recommend you switch to *certified* raw goat's milk (avoid pasteurized goat's milk, which has had many important enzymes destroyed in the pasteurization process). For those with a weight problem, the best solution regarding dairy products is this: Eliminate them.[12]

"But," you may be saying, "I love cheese!" So do I. It was once one of my all-time favorite foods. When I discovered its potential for harm to my heart and cardiovascular system, however, I had little trouble reducing the amount of cheese in my eating plan and using only no-fat cheese. Most people who are intent on losing fat from their body cells find that they cannot lose fat and eat cheese, or consume other milk products, at the same time.

What about ice cream? Not only does ice cream have the fat of milk, but it also is loaded with sugar and synthetic chemicals, some of which are used for a variety of very unhealthful processes: nitrate solvent, paint solvent, rubber cement manufacturing, lice control, plastics, dyes, and egg emulsifiers. I know that asking you to give up ice cream for the rest of your life may be unrealistic. I admit I still have a soft spot for good ice cream and I give in to its temptation once or twice a year. If you must eat ice cream, choose the highest-quality ice cream you can find (which is good advice regarding any dairy product you feel you must eat). I personally recommend Breyers or Haagen-Dazs ice creams because they have no stabilizers, gums, artificial flavors, or toxic additives.

SAY NO TO MARGARINE PRODUCTS

Margarine and all margarine-like products—including most commercially produced peanut butters—are loaded with partially hydrogenated fats or trans fats (some of which we discussed earlier). Two tablespoons of peanut butter has more fat than one tablespoon of pure grease!

Not only is hydrogenated peanut butter high in dangerous fats, but so are other margarine products such as cake icings and candy bars of all types. This fat is what gives these products their "smooth mouth" feel. Many of the thickeners, texturizers, and fillers used in processed foods include these fats because people like the "thick and creamy" feel on their tongue.

If you really want maximum fat loss, you must stay away from all margarine products, polyunsaturated oils, and hydrogenated fats, and use only olive oil or small amounts of organic butter to cook.

Basically, hydrogenated fats are fats that have a very high "burn" temperature and that are firm and white if left at room temperature (canned shortening is an example). Hydrogenated fats are used by fast-food restaurants and are in most processed foods because they are plentiful, cheap, and seem to have a very long shelf life. They are not only very hazardous to human health, but they may very well be the number one cause of many life-threatening diseases that seem epidemic in our culture today. If you look historically at the manufacturing and use of hydrogenated fats, you will find their use in our culture increased shortly before our nation's huge escalation of instances of heart disease and cancers that involve the soft tissues and the digestive tract.

These fats are associated with increased LDL cholesterol (bad cholesterol), coronary heart disease, and breast cancer.[13]

While we're dealing with this area of food products, let me also say a word about Olean and Olestra, the "fake fat" that actually had its beginning as a trial drug meant to control cholesterol. The drug didn't perform very well, so Proctor & Gamble withdrew its application for drug approval and applied for approval of its hybrid fake fat as a food additive. This may be one of the deadliest-ever attempts to fool Mother Nature.

If someone told you to eat a product that has a high likelihood of producing gas, bloody stools, cramps, rectal seepage, and diarrhea, you'd probably say "no, thanks." Well, that's exactly the response you should have to Olestra-laced products. Not only does Olestra have negative side effects, it actually has negative nutritional value because it prevents the body from absorbing carotenoids (which protect against chronic diseases such as cancer and heart disease)."[14]

AND THEN WE COMBINE THE WORST OF THE WORST. . .

and call it pizza! Think about it. Take pork products (pepperoni), milk products (cheese toppings), white flour (crust), and fats, combine them and bake at a high degree to release their maximum toxicity, and what do you get? America's favorite food. As far as I am concerned, pizza is one of the worst fat culprits in our culture. (Ice cream and cheese are two others.)

I recently heard of a person who ordered a half-pepperoni, half-shrimp pizza. He managed to get all of the five worst foods on one plate!

Our church youth group had a party at our house not too long ago, and what did they bring as food? Boxes and boxes of double-decker pizza. I nearly passed out.

Actually, I have been amazed that almost any time I go to a youth function, pizza is served. I am convinced that pizza is the number one reason we have so many fat children and teens in our society today.

I have a home gym. I invited several of the guys in our church youth group to come over and work out with me, in part so I could teach them how to work out safely. One of the boys who came over was extremely overweight, with probably 40 percent body fat. After only one week of working out, this young man had lost eleven pounds. What changes did I ask him to make in his dietary plan? I asked him to do only three things: drink more water, stop eating bread, and stop eating pizza. By the way, he has now lost 43 pounds and 10 inches from his waist in approximately ninety days. Do you think he is excited?

If pizza is placed before you and it's all that is provided for you to eat, choose to eat only the meat, cheese, and vegetable toppings.

Granted, you'll be getting a hefty dose of fat with the protein, but at least you'll be cutting out the carbohydrates from the bread base of the pizza.

I used this trick when I was in college at Florida State. My friends and I would go to The Subway Restaurant there in Tallahassee (not to be confused with today's Subway sandwich shops) and they'd always order double-extra beef and cheese pizza. I'd scrape off the toppings and eat only those. I didn't know all that I know today, but I had observed years earlier as a young athlete that bread made me gain fat very quickly. Over the months my college friends grew fatter and fatter and I stayed thin and in shape. I know part of the reason was my peculiar approach to eating pizza without its crust and of course my work out program.

MAKE YOUR DECISION AT THE GROCERY STORE

The best way to keep the foods identified in this chapter out of your body are to keep them out of your grocery cart. What is kept out of your grocery cart doesn't make it to your kitchen or pantry shelves. And what isn't on your shelves doesn't make it into your body. Make your decision for maximum fat loss at the grocery store, not the dining table. You'll find it much easier to say no at the grocery store. Simply refuse to go up and down certain aisles in the market!

- Eliminate all pork products from your diet.

- No artificial sweeteners!

- Cut out all shellfish.

- Remove all the junk food from your grocery cart.

- Avoid high-fat dairy products.

- Say no to margarine, shortening, and hydrogenated oil products.

- Eliminate all pizza delivery numbers from the memory bank of your telephone!

You may be thinking, *Well, Ted, if I avoid all these products, what can I snack on?* The subject of snacking is next.

10

COPING WITH
THE CRAVINGS

Most of the chronic dieters I have encountered fear one thing: the "craves."

For the most part, food cravings begin in the brain. Generalized feelings of emptiness or hunger are translated in the brain as a desire for a specific food. The more a person dwells on the *idea* of that food, the stronger the craving grows. Cravings have probably sunk more diets than any other single factor.

A craving may be a mental habit. You are used to eating a particular food so your brain thinks you should continue eating it. Each time you successfully overcome a craving, you are helping to build a new brain habit.

Another reason you may be having cravings is low blood sugar and that may be due to a deficiency of some nutrient used in blood sugar regulation. I use a powdered product from my office called Glycemix. This stabilizes my blood sugar cravings. It basically eliminates these types of cravings.

In eating six meals a day, you are not likely to experience any great hunger pangs. At the outset of a fat-loss program, however, some of those "snack attacks" can occur. There are several things you can do to avoid them and, if they occur, to overcome them.

TIPS TO AVOID SNACK ATTACKS

Prevention is always better than either an active defense or offense! Here are specific things you can do to avoid getting a snack attack.

Don't Skip Meals!

This is especially important for breakfast. Skipping a meal sends a signal to your body that you are moving into starvation mode and your body will automatically move to reduce your metabolic rate.

Another danger of skipping a meal is that you will have a strong tendency to binge at a future meal, and often this meal is the last one of the day (which is the very meal during which you should not overeat). Skipping a meal also impairs your body's ability to recover from exercise.

Eat Enough Fiber.

We discuss the specifics about fiber in a later chapter, but for our purposes here you need to know that one of the best curbs for keeping a person from feeling empty is fiber. Fiber not only gives feelings of fullness with less food, but it also improves the stability of blood sugar levels. It works by slowing the movement of food from the stomach to the small intestine. In addition, the body uses more energy—burns up more calories—in absorbing high-fiber foods than low-fiber ones. This is why I use coarse wheat bran in my protein shakes.

Do Not Chew Gum.

It increases the flow of gastric juices that trigger hunger.

Anticipate the Timing of When a Snack Attack Is Likely to Occur.

Some people get into habits of eating specific things at specific times—cheese and crackers at four o'clock, a cookie with tea at five o'clock, or a candy bar as part of a morning work break. Recognize those habits in your life.

Drinking a small amount of a "green food" drink—about an hour before you've usually had a snack food in your old eating pattern—can greatly decrease sugar-craving and binge-eating.

Green foods, such as spirulina, chlorella, and barley green extracts, are nutrient-dense and low-calorie super foods. Many contain generous amounts of amino acids along with essential fatty acids, vitamins, and trace minerals. They can energize you and help curb your food cravings without adding empty calories to an eating plan. These foods are available in powdered form, tablets, and capsules, and are sometimes mixed with other ingredients in many weight-reduction meal replacement products. They can help stave off cravings.[1] Also there are a lot of nutrition bars available on the market that are actually an alternative to eating junk food. Some of them actually taste quite good.

Don't Binge.

I recently read a weight-loss article that suggested that a person give himself permission to "pig out" once a week to avoid "going crazy." The author suggested that a person hold off eating apple pie, french fries, pizza, candy, and other foods until Pig-Out Day and then forget calorie counting, portion control, and nutrition completely on that one day a week. The idea was that this one day of eating whatever you want would give you the discipline to eat the right things the other six days of the week. I don't recommend this approach.

Remember, too many sweets and fats in a day can actually stimulate your craving for those items the second day, and it's almost as if you are back to square one in trying to motivate yourself to maintain a fat-loss program.

Eliminate as Many "Food Cues" as Possible.

Food cures are usually visual images that trigger a desire for a specific food. Most of these cues come via television and billboards. Do you think the advertisers know this?

Just think about all the food commercials that a person sees in just a couple of hours of television viewing. Those commercials are designed to make you hungry. One of the best things you can do for yourself during the first couple of weeks of a fat-loss program is to turn off your television set and choose to either read a book, listen to an inspirational or instructional tape and take notes as you listen, or take a walk—all three of which are probably better for your mind as well as your body!

When driving, listen to tapes and keep your eyes on the road.

For some people, cravings hit the minute they walk into the kitchen or see the refrigerator. If that's true for you, stay out of the kitchen and make sure your kitchen is only stocked with healthy, low-glycemic foods.

When you're at the mall, do your best to avoid the food court—in fact, avoid shopping in areas where food is offered. The aroma alone can trigger a hunger craving.

How do they make those cinnamon buns smell so good? The answer is hydrogenated fat, sugar, and artificial colors and flavorings plus a big fan to blow the aroma into the very path you walk. You may as well paste those cinnamon buns on to your thights, because that's where they are likely to end up. if they don't kill you first with heart disease or cancer.

MAKE A LIST OF ALTERNATIVES TO SNACKING

Make and keep handy a small list of alternative activities to eating. These should be things you can do quickly, easily, and frequently, and ideally be things that you do with your hands. I know one woman who decided that every time she felt a craving for food she would go out into her yard and pull two dozen weeds. After a couple of weeks she found that her cravings were far fewer and her flower beds were virtually weed-free!

Another woman reached for her latest crochet project when she felt a craving. A male client decided that he'd turn his cravings into shoe-polishing time—when he ran out of his own pairs of shoes that needed polishing, he took on all his family's shoes!

Here are ten examples of the many things you might do when a craving strikes:

1. Take a quick walk, even if it's just around the block. (This is not a substitute for your morning aerobic workout. It's a bit of extra exercise to shunt the blood away from your stomach and to put food out of your mind.)

2. Pick up a piece of needlework or handwork, or catch up on your mending.

3. Write a note to a friend that you've been meaning to contact for awhile. Or head for your computer and do a little e-mailing to folks you haven't written to in awhile.

4. Drink a large glass of pure water. Often this is sufficient to satisfy the immediate empty feeling.

5. Consider taking that large glass of water out into your yard. Enjoy the beauty of your garden for a few minutes. (If your garden isn't beautiful, perhaps pull a few weeds, plant a few flowers, rake a few leaves, or mow a little grass!) Perhaps spend a little time in quiet contemplation or prayer in the beauty of the outdoors.

6. Pick up a book or magazine and immerse yourself in it. Concentrate on what you are reading, not on the food you *thought* you needed.

7. Take a shower or soak for ten minutes in your whirlpool tub.

8. Surf the Internet.

9. Polish two pieces of furniture in your house (or clean a window, or polish a mirror or two). You might be amazed at how many household chores you can get done in a short five-minute spurt of effort designed to take your mind off a food craving!

10. Call a friend in your support group and ask that person what he or she does when a craving strikes. Expand your list of options by adopting the strategies of others.

BATTLING THE ATTACK

Food cravings tend to peak and subside like ocean waves. If you get an urge to eat, tell yourself that you can satisfy that craving if you really want to but then wait ten minutes before taking any action. Tell your spouse when you have a craving to be strong for you and you'll be strong for them. Usually the craving will subside in that time. If not, then you have the confidence that your eating is at least a conscious act and not a compulsive act.

Don't just sit at the kitchen table, however, thinking about the food craving for ten minutes! Get up and do something else. Distract yourself.

But remember, don't keep that item in the house. Force yourself to get dressed, get in your car, drive to the store—and perhaps by the time you get to the store you will have come to your senses, laugh about your craving, and drive back home. Above all, do not buy more than you can eat. Buying an item in quantity solely because it is cheaper by the dozen or gallon is a bad idea—this leaves excess food around to be converted into excess fat!

Reach for Pen and Paper.

When you feel hunger between meals, which isn't all that likely if you are eating six meals a day, try reaching for a pen and paper instead of food. Write down what you believe triggered your craving. Analyze the craving. Is the craving more emotional or physical? Could the craving be satisfied without food? In writing out your response to hunger, you become much more aware of what triggers hunger. In making this discovery, you can usually isolate what to avoid. You also become aware that much of what we call *hunger* actually has little to do with a physical need for food.

I recently heard about one woman who kept a "hunger notepad" with her at all times. She discovered that the chiming of her grandfather clock seemed to signal in her a feeling that it was time to eat—every time the clock struck twelve, she headed for the kitchen, and every time the clock struck six, she also sought out food. She said, "I was just like Pavlov's dogs—ring that bell and I started salivating."

Her solution? She stopped the chiming of the clock and stopped wearing a watch. Instead, she set her wrist watch to sound a little alarm at the appropriate times for her to eat a meal. It took about three months, but she gradually reprogrammed her body so that she automatically knew when it was time for a meal.

As part of noting your response to hunger pangs, you might also write down your own answers to questions such as the ones below—take on only one question each time you feel hungry. You can learn a lot about yourself, and what has motivated your eating in the past if you answer these questions honestly:

- What do you consider to be "too fat"?

- In what ways has being overweight caused you emotional pain?

- Is there any limitation you have experienced that you believe is caused by your weight?

- Have you used food as a reward, punishment, obligation, or substitute for love?

- What were your favorite childhood foods?

- Is it more important to you to look good or feel good?

- When you see overweight people, what do you think about them?

- What makes you feel guilty? (Be specific.)

- In what ways have you used your weight as an excuse for not doing certain things?

- Is there something you'd really like to do but don't think you can do as long as you are overfat?

- Is there someone other than yourself that you are trying to please by losing fat? (or are you really losing fat to please yourself?)

- What are you first food memories?

- What emotions have you attached to mealtimes in the past?

- Are all of your emotional and spiritual needs being met? If not, what can you do to meet those needs apart from eating?

- Do you tell yourself lies about what you eat or how much you eat?

- Do you lie to yourself about exercise?

- Are you making healthy choices regarding your work and your social life?

- Do your food attitudes parallel your attitudes toward love, money, and sex?

- What words come to mind when you hear these words: party, festivity, celebration?

- What words come to your mind when you hear the word exercise?

Also consider making a list of things you intend to do once you have lost weight. Then, pick out one thing from that list and do it every week of your fat-loss plan or after the loss of every five pounds of fat.

Put on a Tight Belt.

One of the easiest and simplest strategies for dealing with a snack attack is to go to your closet and put on a tight belt, or tighten your belt several notches until it is tight. That tight belt will remind you that you are *intent* on losing excess fat from your body!

Make Good Choices.

Here are some good choices to make to drive away the hunger and also add the right kinds of foods to your eating plan:

- Celery and carrot sticks. I suggest you prepare a batch of these at the beginning of the week and keep them in airtight baggies so they are readily available for snack attacks.

- Fat-free cottage cheese topped with homemade or fresh applesauce (without any preservative) and a few walnuts. This can actually be a meal in itself!

- Unsweetened gelatin made with natural fruit juice in place of the sugar and water recommended on most gelatin boxes.

- A slice of watermelon, a piece of fresh fruit, or a frozen fruit Popsicle made from natural fruit juice.

- Fat-free yogurt topped with a few nuts or a piece of fresh fruit. Again, this can be an entire small meal.

- Herbal teas mixed with very diluted (10:1 ratio) unsweetened fruit juice. These are a satisfying low-calorie drink and are also very filling.

- Sparkling water mixed with very diluted (10:1 ratio) natural fruit juice in place of a soda. Sip your beverages slowly. And limit your intake of sparkling water—many of these water products are high in sodium. These also decrease the oxygen in the bloodstream.

- My wife also has great ideas in her cookbook.

THIS, TOO, SHALL PASS

Over time, you will probably feel fewer and fewer cravings. If cravings persist and they seem to be at a particular time of day, consider adjusting the timing of one or more of your meals.

Consider giving yourself a reward for overcoming a set number of craving attacks. Remind yourself that each time you withstand an attack you are doing something positive for both your body and your mind. In a phrase, *you are taking control!*

Do not go to a grocery store when you are hungry or just before a meal. There are way too many food cues for you to battle. Go to the grocery store when you feel full and satisfied, and ideally only once a week.

Speaking of the grocery store, there are specific strategies that can help you with shopping, cooking, and dining out. We go there next.

11

TIPS FOR SHOPPING, COOKING, AND EATING OUT

Do you remember when the cereal at the grocery store was found in an aisle that also shelved several other food products? Not anymore! That cereal aisle is an aisle all to itself, with top-to-bottom shelving for all kinds of cereal products.

Do you remember when a few boxes of macaroni and spaghetti were the sum total of the pasta offerings in a supermarket? Not today! You'll find dozens of pasta-based products.

The same goes for cookies, crackers, and a host of other snack foods and prepackaged foods. The candy bar display runs for several linear feet and the ice cream section can also be an aisle unto itself. The two or three frozen TV dinners that once appeared tucked into a meat freezer have expanded until there dozens and dozens of frozen meals to choose from, most of them very high in calories with pasta and grain products as their base.

Your first battlefront in winning the war against fat is going to be in your local supermarket.

STRATEGIES FOR WISE GROCERY SHOPPING

If I could make only one suggestion to you about grocery shopping it would be this: Get your paper products and other nonfood products first and then head straight for the fruits and vegetables area of the supermarket. Load up your cart there and leave a little room for lean meat, poultry, and fish. Then head for the check-out stand, with blinders to the rest of the store! Consider it a rare excursion to check out any other aisle.

Shop From a List.

After you have decided what you are going to eat as your basic meals in any given week, make a shopping list.

First, write down all the things you need for the week. Be sure to include condiments and other supplies. You may need to divide this list into two—things you can purchase at a regular supermarket and things that you need to pick up at a health food or nutrition store.

Second, check your cupboards and pantry. Check off those things you already have in sufficient quantity for the week.

Third, be sure to go to the store with your list in hand. Stick to your list. Don't let your cart wander into aisles that don't have items you need. Don't let your eyes stray from the immediate things you are purchasing! Advertisers are excellent at getting you to buy a product that you don't need. It is almost a war in which they want to take you prisoner and force you to do their will. Don't give in to their demands. Avoid them like the plague.

Don't Shop Hungry.

Don't go to the story hungry. Period. It is better to go home and have a meal than to stop at the store on your way home from work and purchase all the wrong things!

RETHINK YOUR KITCHEN AND COOKING STRATEGIES

Conduct a basic inventory of your own kitchen. Do you have the cookware you need?

- Do you have a nonstick pan?
- Do you have a juicer for making your own fruit and vegetable juices from fresh produce?
- Do you have a blender for making protein drinks?
- Do you have a scale for weighing portions of meat and grains?
- Do you have a grain grinder for preparing your own whole-grain flour?

Certainly you don't *need* these appliances, but they make cooking more convenient and nutritious.

Check your pantry too. Simply throw out those things that you know aren't good for you. Why keep on hand things that will tempt you to snack or that you know are doing more harm than good to your body?

Ten Smart-Cooking Tips

Here are ten tips that are easy to incorporate into your cooking routines and that can make a significant difference:

1. Use small amounts of olive oil spray.

2. Use water or a little vegetable or chicken broth rather than sautéing with oil or butter. One cup of chicken stock has only about twenty calories, while one tablespoon of oil has 120 calories. Vegetable juice and apple cider vinegar can also be used for sautéing. You will need to watch your pan more closely and stir often, though, since these non-oil alternatives tend to evaporate more quickly.

3. Use steaming racks for both vegetables and fish. Don't over-steam your foods.

4. Eat more foods that don't require coking. Cooking begins the breakdown of complex carbohydrates. When your body is forced to do that initial breakdown, more calories are required by the digestion process.

5. Drain canned vegetables to get rid of as much of the sodium as possible. Steam your canned vegetables rather than boil them. Boiling only causes more nutrients to be lost. Remember canned veggies are one of the worst choices. Always try to buy fresh or frozen.

6. Consider preparing several portions of chicken or fish at the same time and freezing the unused portions. This makes meal-preparation easier at later meals. It's just as easy to microwave a premade portion of food that is good for you as it is to reach for a fast-food snack that isn't good for you!

7. Always season foods at the table, not as part of the cooking process. Try putting unusual spices on the table rather than the salt shaker.

8. Don't taste your cooking unless absolutely necessary. It's amazing how many calories you can consume by just tasting a sauce or dish several times before it is done. Plus, when you taste there is no way to log the amount of calories you are consuming.

9. Make a homemade stew, chili, or soup the day before you intend to eat it. Refrigerate the cooked mixture overnight. This allows you to skim off the fat completely before reheating the dish. The flavors of the ingredients will also have a time to mix and the concoction will actually grow in flavor.

10. Use non-fat cheese.

For a surprising number of people, the most difficult food they have to give up on a fat-loss plan is cheese. If you are preparing a dish that *must* have cheese, you can de-fat it by zapping an ounce of it in the microwave for two minutes (on high setting). The fat part of the cheese will liquefy and form a pool on top of the cheese. Pour it off. This method will reduce the amount of fat in one ounce of cheese by about four grams. This method works best with mozzarella and cheddar cheeses.

One note: Always stay at least eight feet away from a microwave when it is turned on. Microwave ovens put out a lot of electromagnetic energy, which can be dangerous.

GIVE YOURSELF A NEW TASTE SENSATION

One of the problems many people on a fat-loss program seem to complain about is monotony in their food choices. People seem to become bored with eating foods that are good for them. Part of the reason is that they have failed to be creative in their food choices. They limit themselves to only a few items and then leave these unseasoned.

Be creative.

Be creative in your eating. Most Americans aren't.

Are you aware that the average American eats only about twenty different foods a week? Most people have become dietary drones. They eat the same thing just about every day with very few variations. Try some new taste sensations as part of your fat-loss program. Make losing fat a creative venture that also translates into gaining taste sophistication!

If you're in the produce section of the grocery store and you don't know the name of a particular fruit or vegetable, ask the grocer responsible for that area. Most of them would love to educate a customer—not only on the name and nature of the food item, but also on ways to prepare it.

Try some new recipes. I suggest you consult a cookbook for recipes only after you have eaten. Consider the recipe for your *next* meal a couple of hours away, or for a meal the next day or next week.

Think variety when it comes to your meal plans. Try new foods. Don't get stuck in a rut eating the same thing every day.

Experiment with condiments

Condiments are great for giving a good taste variety to a fat-loss eating plan. Experiment with the following:

- fresh garlic
- bay leaves
- allspice
- cinnamon
- cloves
- tumeric
- cayenne pepper
- curry powder

- low-salt defatted broths
- fresh salsa
- ¼ cup pumpkin seeds
- ⅛ cup walnuts
- various types of flavored peppers (key lime, lemon)
- do not use MSG

Try spices such as curry or saffron for an added zing. Visit an Asian market or a Middle Eastern market and ask about the various spices you find. Try a couple of them for yourself!

Try flavored vinegars as a condiment for your salads. You can get a lot of flavor for relatively few calories.

Japanese tamari or shoyu can be substituted for high-sodium soy sauce. (Watch out for MSG! Most soy sauce is loaded with it.)

Nutmeg, ginger, and mustard can enhance the flavor of just about all foods from eggs to vegetables to meats to whole grains.

Rather than use salt, try lemon juice or vinegar. Try putting lemon juice in a spritzer or food atomizer. Just a spritz of lemon can add a lot of flavor to a plate of lightly steamed vegetables.

FIVE TABLESIDE EATING TIPS

Meal Companions

You tend to weigh about the same amount that your friends weigh. Think about it. If your friends are overweight, you are more likely to be overweight. Why? First, you tend to eat what they eat when you are with them. And second, overweight friends give you a certain comfort zone about your weight. If you eat with people who have poor eating habits and who give a green light to your excess fat, you aren't going to be very motivated to stick to a maximum fat-loss eating plan.

Am I advocating that you give up friendships? Not necessarily. Just don't *eat* with your overweight friends. And do your best to encourage at least one or more of your friends to join you in pursuing a maximum fat-loss program. This way you can encourage one another to continue in your program until you reach your goals.

Small Plates

Consider using small plates for your meals. Bread-and-butter plates or salad plates can look like a "full plate of food."

Intentional Eating

Pay close attention to every bite you put into your mouth.

One of the unwritten laws of the universe is this: Don't fall asleep when you're behind the wheel. Millions of people, however, seem to fall asleep mentally as soon as they sit down to eat. They shovel things into their mouth without any awareness of what they are eating or how much they are eating.

"It was only a few chips." In reality, if you had been counting, it was *thirty-eight* chips.

"I didn't have second helpings of *everything*." No, in reality, you had second helpings only of mashed potatoes, gravy, meatloaf, and a second roll.

"I can't remember what I had for dinner last night." No, because you were watching TV at the same time you shoveled in three pieces of leftover pizza, drank a large cola, and ate the rest of the chocolate cream pie.

"It was only one scoop of ice cream." In reality, it was a scoop of ice cream that filled the entire cereal bowl.

A Large Glass of Water

Drink a glass of purified water before you take your first bite of a meal. Then drink another large glass after you finish your meal.

Eating Slowly

Thoroughly chew your food. A good trick to slow your eating is to set your fork down between each bite and not pick it up again until you have thoroughly chewed and swallowed what is in your mouth and followed it with a sip of water.

DEFATTING YOUR RESTAURANT EXPERIENCES

Choose to eat out less. A recent survey revealed that about half of all adult Americans eat more meals out than at home! Cut down on your dining out. You'll face far fewer temptations to binge or to eat the wrong foods.

As much as possible, know in advance of going to a restaurant or fast-food place exactly what you intend to order. Then, don't even pick up the menu. Menus are written and illustrated to tempt you to buy as much food as possible, generally with the highest caloric content. Those full-color photographs are better avoided!

Refuse to be enticed by what others with you may order. As much as possible, choose to order first. That way you will be less tempted to change your order to comply with the gooey, calorie-laden items others may be choosing.

Do you have to give up every restaurant dish you have grown to love? Consider the suggestions below if you are in a restaurant or at a party:

- Instead of potato chips . . . choose carrot sticks.
- Instead of fried foods . . . choose baked or grilled.
- Instead of breaded foods . . . choose unbreaded.
- Instead of "two large scoops" or "two large serving spoons" of anything . . . go for one small scoop or spoonful.
- Instead of a twelve-ounce T-bone . . . choose a twelve-ounce fish filet.

- Instead of a baked potato . . . choose other side vegetables that are low on the glycemic scale.

- Instead of eating Mexican food three times a week . . . have a low-fat Mexican dish once every two weeks.

- Instead of smothering a salad with high-calorie salad dressing . . .choose a nonfat vinaigrette with extra wedges of lemon and ground pepper and ask for all of these items to be served on the side. Two tablespoons of regular salad dressing— which is about the amount in the average restaurant salad-bar ladle—contain about two hundred calories. Two tablespoons of hot fudge sauce have fewer calories and a lot less fat! Use salad dressing sparingly, perhaps even only on every third or fourth bite.

- Look for low-fat, low-calorie, and heart-healthy items on a menu. Especially look for an explanation that tells you how many calories or fat grams these options have.

- Order everything à la carte. Sometimes soup and salad can be a meal—the same for salad and an appetizer.

- Ask for extra steamed vegetables rather than the potato or rice or pasta that comes with many meals.

- Order grilled or baked foods rather than fried. Even if the menu lists only fried, ask that the chef grill your choice. Especially avoid deep-fried or breaded-and-fried foods. Don't be fooled by the phrase "lightly sautéed." That's still a form of frying!

- Order any sauces (such as hollandaise) to be served on the side or left off.

- Split a meal. Consider splitting an entree or large salad with someone else at your table. Simply ask for a second plate and do the dividing yourself. This is what my wife and I do every time we go out. You can split meals at home as well. One of the best ways to eat six meals a day is simply to divide the three meals you would normally eat and space out your consumption.

- Ask for a "lunch portion." Many menus now have the option of a "lunch size" or "dinner size" entrée.
- If you are eating by yourself, eat only half of what you are served. When you order your meal, ask your waiter for a take-home box. Divide your meal in half even before you take the first bite. (In some cases, you may want to store two-thirds of the meal for two small meals later. In fact, given the huge portions served at some restaurants these days, you may want to box up three-quarters of the meal for three small meals later. This can make eating out more economical as well as better for fat loss.)

A Party Tip

If you going to a party, bring a small toothbrush in your purse or pocket. Excuse yourself to the bathroom and brush your teeth after you know you've had your calorie limit. You'll be less apt to reach for another bite after you've brushed your teeth.

When Flying

If you are traveling by air, call your airline twenty-four hours before takeoff to order a special meal. Ask for "pure-vegetarian, no-oil" meals or a fruit plate. You can always put some fresh-vegetable snacks in a baggie and carry them on board in your purse or carry-on luggage.

EATING OUT AT FAST-FOOD SPOTS

Do you need to cut out all fast-food stops on a fat-loss plan? Not necessarily.

If you find yourself with no alternative but a fast-food spot, make sure you only choose *one* item and eat it slowly. Choose an item that has grilled or roasted chicken—no breading, no deep-fat frying. Grilled chicken is great on a salad with nonfat vinaigrette dressing.

Ask for any "special sauce" to be omitted. The same goes for all mayo or cheese. Choose mustard or a fat-free dressing. (Mustard is better than ketchup—ketchup is loaded with sugar.)

If your one food item is something like a grilled chicken burrito, you can spice it up with mild or hot sauce (salsa or pico de gallo). You can also add zip to just about any salad or food item with jalapeños or pickles.

Some delis offer whole chicken breasts or slices of turkey breast. If side orders are available, look for steamed vegetables or fruit salad.

Ask for lots of lettuce and tomato on the side. It's worth any extra fee they might charge you.

Make sure all the skin has been removed from chicken or turkey. If you have your choice between white and dark meat, choose white.

If you're at a fish place, make sure the fish is baked, not breaded or fried.

WHAT YOU DON'T EAT CAN'T HURT YOU!

Remind yourself often that what you don't put into your mouth can't hurt you. What you don't put into your shopping cart can't be cooked or eaten at home. Prevention is a part of fat-loss!

Also keep this in the forefront of your thinking any time you start to feel deprived of a once-favorite food or dish: Nothing tastes as good as being in great shape feels! This is a great slogan to write out and put on your refrigerator door.

Food isn't the only thing you put into your body, of course. What you drink can be just as important as what you eat. That's next.

KEY #7:

**Drink half your weight in ounces of
pure water every day.**

12

WHAT YOU DRINK CAN BE JUST AS IMPORTANT AS WHAT YOU EAT

Any person on a fat-loss program has a great friend and ally in pure water.

Many people I've met through the years have an erroneous idea that water consumption results in added "water weight." The exact opposite is true.

Water is a natural diuretic. When water is adequately supplied to the body, a signal goes from brain to body that the body does not need to *store* water. That allows the continual flushing of the body to continue, washing away fat globules and other cellular debris from the bloodstream into the urinary tract on a regular and even-flowing basis.

Drinking enough water is critical for maintaining healthy muscle cells. Muscle cells that are deprived of sufficient fluids shrink like a plum that's been left out in the sun too long. Shriveled and dehydrated, prunelike muscle cells are no longer capable of optimal growth.

How much water should you drink? Drink half of your body weight in ounces of distilled or reverse-osmosis water every day.

OUR NEED FOR PURER WATER

A number of years ago, *Dragnet*—a popular television program—featured a character who was prone to say, "Just the facts, ma'am." This detective wanted just the facts and nothing but the facts.

When it comes to your water, that's also what you want—just the water, and none of the toxic poisons that so routinely seem to be found in our public drinking water.

Two of the most toxic substances found in our water supply are chlorine and fluoride.

During my college chemistry years, whenever we combined chemicals in the lab that had a potential for releasing chlorine gas, we had to use a vacuum hood to pull the gas out of the lab. We knew that a good inhalation of chlorine gas could send us to the hospital, or worse. It's no secret that chlorine gas has been used as a chemical weapon in past wars.

Even knowing this about chlorine, since World War I we have massively introduced chlorination to our community water supplies as a cheap and effective way to stop some of the epidemics carried by water. By 1940, about a third of the drinking water in the United States was chlorinated, and at present, about seven out of every ten Americans drinks chlorinated water from public water supplies.[1]

Not only can chlorine gas be dangerous in its own right, but chlorination of drinking water has been linked to a number of cancers. When chlorine reacts with organic contaminants, such as dead leaves or other organic residue, it forms by-products called trihalomethanes that are carcinogenic.

Apart from the health hazards of chlorination, chlorinated water can leave a person's skin and hair dry and frayed.

This is a book about maximum fat loss, however, so we must ask the question, "Does chlorination have anything to do with fat in the body?" Yes!

Continual exposure to chlorine can increase your risk of atherosclerotic plaquing because chlorine elevates LDL (bad) cholesterol and suppresses HDL (good) cholesterol. It should not be any surprise that the areas of our nation that have the highest levels of chlorine in their public-water supplies also have the highest numbers of heart-disease patients![2]

Fluoride is chlorine's evil twin sister. It is a by-product of aluminum.

Now both aluminum and fluoride are found in abundance in the plant kingdom (in colloidal form) and in that form, neither is harmful to the body. However, when our bodies come into contact with the metallic form of aluminum, they go berserk. Fluoride acts like rat poison in the body; it accumulates in the glands and fat tissues over time, and is especially prone to accumulation in the thyroid gland. Aluminum has the deadly and devastating ability to move through the brain barrier and do brain damage.

In poison manuals, fluoride is considered to be more toxic than lead and only slightly less toxic than arsenic! Think about that before you brush your teeth again with a fluoride toothpaste.

Fluoride was added to city water supplies in the 1940s because naturally occurring fluoride in the water supply of one Texas town seemed to be the reason that the town's citizens had a lower incidence of dental cavities. Later studies failed to show that fluoride added to water supplies have any effect in preventing dental decay. In fact, studies in recent years have shown fluoride added to water supplies has a carcinogenic effect. Still, fluoride is routinely added to many city water supplies and it is a common ingredient in toothpaste and mouthwash.

Fluoride is so acidic that it severely corrodes lead pipes, lead pipe joint solders, and almost any metal in general. When one city shut down its fluoridation pumps for repairs, they noticed a 78-percent decrease in the amount of lead in their tap water. That should give you pause the next time you turn on the kitchen faucet!

The only way to avoid chlorination and fluoridation in tap water is to use a "reverse osmosis" or steam-distillation water purifier. A variety of units are available at reasonable prices. If you are unable to locate any in your area contact my office for more information. Carbon-block filters do not remove fluoride.[3]

Ask questions. If your community fluoridates its water, don't drink it. Stop using fluoride toothpaste, fluoride drops, or fluoride vitamins.

Any person who is pursuing a maximum fat loss program needs to be washing his or her body—bloodstream, digestive system, and cells—with pure water. That's the best means of transporting both fat and toxins from the body. Don't drink water that *adds* toxins to the body. Those toxins can interact with fat globules in very harmful ways.

Water, Not Water-Based Beverages

A number of people have come to me through the years telling me that they don't enjoy the taste of water. I can understand that. The reason they don't enjoy water's taste is probably because of the chemicals that have been added to the water supply they are tapping. The alternative is to purify your drinking water.

What these people tend to tell me next is just as disturbing to me: They are turning to other beverages thinking that because these beverages are liquid and have a water base, they are good substitutes for water. The common culprits are these three types of beverages:

- caffeine drinks, including coffee, tea, and colas

- alcoholic beverages

- fruit juices and fruit-flavored drinks

Let's deal with these one at a time.

DRINKING COFFEE DOESN'T COUNT

The most widely used drug in our society today is caffeine. It shows up in everything from coffee, tea, chocolate, and cola drinks to aspirin, analgesics, and over-the-counter stimulants. It quickly stimulates the human brain, nervous system, and adrenal glands. It is highly addictive and readily available.

The reason most people seem to turn to coffee or caffeine-laced drinks is because they feel a need for energy, not because they are trying to increase their liquid consumption. Fatigue is a signal to your body that you need to stimulate your body for energy by changing something in your diet. Stimulant drinks don't really solve the fatigue problem.[4]

Americans literally spend billions of dollars a year on caffeine, nicotine, and a variety of other stimulants. It's a little ironic, therefore, that more than half of the American adult population also complains that they suffer from "general fatigue." You'd think by now we would have figured out that stimulants don't do what we hope they will do! My book *Maximum Energy* tells you how to increase your energy levels without stimulants.

A lean, healthy person has more than an ample supply of energy for bodily functions, tissue repair, and a surplus that can be used for outside activities such as work, hobbies, and exercise.

Caffeine has zero calories. How, then, does it impact the fat-loss equation? In one simple and very powerful way: Caffeine stimulates the adrenal system, causing glucose or blood sugar that is stored in the liver to be released in mass quantities into the system. When the cells cannot use this glucose immediately, the excess is stored as fat. If you are going to drink caffeine regardless of what I say, then make sure you do so on an empty stomach before a workout. That way you can burn the extra calories released.

Caffeine consumption has also been associated with an increase in blood fats or triglycerides, known as hypertriglyceridemia.[5]

Not only can caffeine lead to hypoglycemia, low blood sugar, irregular blood-sugar patterns, and adrenal overload, but the tannic acid in most caffeinated drinks interferes with iron and calcium absorption. Caffeine has been linked to gastritis and heartburn. It promotes sleeplessness and irritability. It acts as a diuretic. It has been linked to an increased risk of fibroid-tumor formation in breast tissue. And in high enough concentrations, it has the potential for causing birth defects in unborn children. Those with hypertension who are trying to keep their blood pressure under control—which includes many who are obese—should avoid all caffeinated beverages.

Caffeine robs the body of a great deal and gives back no nutritional substances.

I have some personal experience with all of this. At one point in my life I was totally and completely addicted to caffeinated coffee. I drank eighteen cups a day. I'd set my fully loaded coffeemaker to come on thirty minutes before I got up so I could awaken to the smell of freshly perked coffee. Not that I cared for the taste of coffee—I really didn't like it all that much.

I'd fill my six-cup porcelain Swiss stein almost to the brim and add whole milk and sweeteners. Then I'd sit back and wait for the results to kick in. Another six-cup stein's worth of my "liquid drug" was taken after lunch and a third round was consumed in the evening. It didn't take too many years of this routine before my body was in adrenal exhaustion. I eventually weaned myself off caffeine by reducing my cup intake by one cup a day until I eventually got down to one cup of coffee a day.

I managed to avoid the headaches many people experience with caffeine withdrawal until I got down to that one cup, and then I hit a plateau. My solution was to dilute that cup with milk by one-eighth of a cup a day. (By the way, don't use artificial creamers—they are loaded with hydrogenated oil and sugars.) Finally I reached the place where I was drinking one-eighth of a cup of coffee and almost a full cup of milk! This went on for several weeks.

Even after I weaned myself off caffeine, I did not fully regain my energy level for months. It took that long for my body to purge itself of all the caffeine and high-fat dairy products (as well as the Sudafeds

I had taken on a daily basis for years and years). I go into more detail about caffeine and how it contributed to my heart disease in my book *Maximum Energy*.

For some, caffeine consumption is not linked to coffee or tea, but to cola drinks or large quantities of chocolate. Caffeine in whatever form is still caffeine.

SAY NO TO ALCOHOL

Alcohol is a drug that has a devastating effect on nearly every major system in the human body—and in human society. In the battle against fat, it is a supreme enemy because it radically raises blood sugar levels.

When the *whole* truth is told about alcohol, there is no good value of alcohol to the human body.

Oh, I know that some of the recent news reports have indicated a link between red wine and the lowering of heart disease. This is actually old news. A research study released in 1977 concluded that the residents of France had a lower incidence of heart disease because they drank red wine. Subsequent research has revealed is that the *grape* extract chemical in the wine—an extract that is a powerful antioxidant—is what aids in preventing heart disease. Those who advocate red wine consumption fail to consider the fact that the French have some of the highest incidences of pancreatic cancer, liver cancer, cirrhosis of the liver, and alcoholism. Some cases of osteoporosis and breast cancer are also caused by alcohol consumption.

What the advocates of red wine also fail to note in most cases is that the French eat fewer snack foods and more vegetables, fish, whole grains, and other complex carbohydrates than Americans. They consume only half as much milk as Americans. And most importantly, the French eat only one-eighteenth of the sugar that Americans eat! They also eat only about half of the fruit we eat, which gives them a lower consumption of the fruit sugar fructose.

In addition, the French tend not to use hydrogenated oils such as margarine and shortening—they tend to use real butter, which doesn't cause nearly as many health problems.

Alcohol has been directly linked to obesity in study after study. It only provides empty calories with no nutrients. And very importantly, it suppresses the body's ability to burn fat. Dean Ornish, M.D., has written that:

> When you drink alcohol, your body burns up fat much more slowly than usual. In one study, for example, researchers found that three ounces of alcohol reduced the body's ability to burn fat by about *one-third*. So it is not just the calories and the fact that alcohol is converted into simple sugars that make it fattening, but also the way that alcohol throws off your body's normal disposal of fat in your diet.[6]

In another study, as little as one ounce of alcohol consumed daily decreased the body's ability to burn fat by up to 30 percent! The alcohol was shown to inhibit the production of lipase, the enzyme that burns fat.[7]

Alcohol not only inhibits the burning of fat from fat deposits. It also can interfere with your judgment, including your judgment about what to eat! After a couple of drinks, you may find yourself eating things you ordinarily would not eat and would not even crave! Better to eliminate alcohol altogether.

CHECK THE FRUIT JUICE LABELS

Fruit *drinks* are not at all the same as fruit *juice*. Some so-called fruit drinks actually have 10 percent or less actual fruit juice. They are little more than fruit-flavored, sugar-loaded water.

"But what about diet drinks?" you may be asking. We'll turn to that important topic next.

13

SURPRISE—NOT *ALL* DIET FOODS ARE GOOD FOR YOU!

Several years ago a man came to advise me on the fence I wanted to put around our property. I noticed that he didn't look particularly well. I asked him if he was having health problems and he told me he was doing okay but he had been through brain surgery the previous year.

"Why did you need brain surgery?" I asked.

He replied, "I was having multiple seizures every day and I had developed a hole in the frontal lobe of my brain. The surgeon had to go in and tie off the blood vessels in that area."

I asked him, "Were you drinking diet sodas?"

He turned as pale as a sheet of paper and said, "How did you know that?"

I said, "Well, I recently came across a research study in which every monkey that was used in an aspartame study developed grand mal epileptic seizures. In another study, half of the animals died after they were given regular doses of aspartame.

He said, "Ted, let me tell you what happened to me. I went to a neurologist after I started experiencing seizures. He tried to induce a seizure while I was in his office and hooked up to various machines. Nothing he tried worked. Finally the neurologist walked in with a diet soda and said, 'Here, drink this. Diet sodas seem to cause seizures in a number of my patients.' I drank the soda, and within five minutes I had a massive seizure."

Mark had never had difficulty with seizures prior to his starting to drink diet sodas. The surgery he had was very difficult because it involved tying off blood vessels that seemed to be "dangling" in holes that had developed in his brain tissue. It was only by the grace of God that he survived. By the way, aspartic acid, a component of aspartame, has been shown to cause holes to develop in brain tissue.

My friend Howard did not survive.

Howard was a good friend of our family and he took me under his wing when I was a young teenager. He taught me the importance of getting good grades and going to college. He was the first person to really emphasize to me the importance of the decisions and choices I made as a teenager. Howard had a good job as a chemist, drove a nice car, and lived in a nice house, so I looked up to him and took his words to heart. He was a real mentor to me.

Several years ago I saw Howard and he told me with tears in his eyes that he had been diagnosed with four inoperable malignant brain tumors, which is usually a death sentence.

I asked him, "Have you been drinking a lot of aspartame products?" He told me that he used NutraSweet in his coffee and tea and that was basically all he drank all day.

I also asked him, "Do you eat a lot of cured meats, such as bacon and other luncheon meats?"

"Every day," he said. He was a man who routinely had bacon and eggs for breakfast and a sandwich made with luncheon-meat for lunch.

I told him that a number of researchers were looking at a possible link between NutraSweet and the nitrates found in luncheon meats and brain cancer. I told him I wanted to contact Dr. John Olney, who is considered by many to be the number one neuropathologist in the world. Dr. Olney was even interviewed on the T.V. show *60 Minutes* about this very topic.

While there was nothing that Dr. Olney could recommend for my friend, Howard, I did learn a great deal from him. I feel compelled by both my friend's death and what I've learned to share this information with you.

Last year I spoke at a seminar held at the Omni in Atlanta. About seventeen thousand people were present. During my presentation I asked the crowd, "How many of you have had a friend, relative, or job acquaintance who has been diagnosed with or has died of a brain tumor?" I was shocked. Almost every person in the Omni raised his or her hand! Perhaps many of you have also had a similar experience or maybe you are wondering why you are hearing so much about brain cancer in the media. Read on for some thought-provoking answers.

SOUNDING THE ALARM ABOUT ASPARTAME

Many people who embark on a fat-loss program turn to diet foods and diet sodas, as well as to the little blue packets of sweetener found on virtually every restaurant table in the land.

As far as I am concerned, aspartame is more dangerous to you than excess fat.

Aspartame appears under many registered names: NutraSweet, Equal, and Spoonful are three of the most common.

Aspartame is used in more than nine thousand products on the market today. It is found in

- instant breakfast drinks
- tabletop sweeteners
- cereals
- sugar-free chewing gum
- instant teas and coffees
- cocoa mixes

- frozen desserts
- flavored coffee and tea beverages
- protein drink powders
- puddings
- gelatin desserts
- juice beverages
- soft drinks
- laxatives
- some multivitamins
- breath mints
- milk drinks
- sugar-free yogurt
- some pharmaceuticals
- wine coolers
- topping mixes
- breakfast cereals

Any time you are looking at a product that claims to be "sugar-free," check the label for aspartame.

Although aspartame is very sweet, roaches won't eat it, cats and dogs won't touch it, ants avoid it, and flies fly the other way from it. The American public, however, flocks to it.

What Is Aspartame and What Happens to It in the Body?

Aspartame was discovered by accident in 1965 when a chemist of the G. D. Searle Company, James Schlatter, was testing an antiulcer drug. He found that a by-product of his experiment tasted very "sweet" and had a "clean" taste without any bitter aftertaste (such as with saccharin). The product was named "Aspartame."

When you combine diketopiperuzine (DKP) and nitrites you have the potential of forming a nitrusurea. Nitrusureas are the most effective agents known for producing malignant brain tumors in laboratory animals. So, if you eat luncheon meat, pepperoni, bacon, ham, or anything with nitrites and then drink a diet soda, or glass of tea or coffee sweetened with aspartame, you have just given your body the raw materials needed to form the most potent brain cancer causing agent known to man. How many folks do you know who eat pepperoni pizza and chase it down with a diet soda?

In the body, aspartame breaks down into the chemicals methanol, aspartic acid, phenylalanine, and diketopiperazine (DKP). Each of these component parts is, by itself, a known toxin!

Methanol, also known as wood alcohol, breaks down into formaldehyde and formic acid. The effects of this one substance alone can cause lethargy, fainting, headaches, nausea, vomiting, blindness, coughing, breathing difficulties, and vision problems. To put things into perspective, just one little blue packet of sweetener (one gram) breaks down into one hundred milligrams of methanol.

Researchers have shown that a child who consumes less than three-fourths of one little blue packet is ingesting almost ten times the Environmental Protection Agency's (EPA) recommended daily limit of methanol consumption for a child. The results are even worse if the product has been exposed to heat or has been on the shelf for a long time.[1]

Free methanol begins to form in liquid aspartame-containing products at temperatures above 86 degrees Fahrenheit. The human body, of course, runs at around 98.6 degrees Fahrenheit. Once ingested, the free methanol is released into the small intestine and encounters the enzyme chymotrypsin, which breaks the methanol down into formaldehyde—yes, the embalming fluid.

The body has difficulty eliminating formaldehyde so it combines some of it with water and stores it in the fat. What is not stored in the fat is further converted to formic acid (which is used as an activator to strip epoxy and urethane coatings—powerful stuff to be floating around among human cells).

Phenylalanine and aspartic acid—90 percent of aspartame—are amino acids normally used in the synthesis of proteoplasm when they are found naturally in foods. When they are unaccompanied by the other amino acids present in natural food sources, they move past the blood-brain barrier and deteriorate the neurons of the brain. The phenylalanine is what breaks down into diketopiperazine (DKP).

A dieter's empty stomach accelerates all of these conversions and amplifies the damage to the body and brain.

The Growing Medical Evidence of Aspartame-Related Disease.

Current literature seems to indicate that each of these diseases could be triggered by aspartame: brain tumors, lupus, Alzheimer's, chronic fatigue, multiple sclerosis, Graves' disease, epilepsy, infertility, Parkinson's disease, lymphoma, Epstein-Barr, psychosis, fibromyalgia, retardation, miscarriages, tremors, infant death, diabetes, breast tumors, and Lou Gehrig's disease.

Here are just some of the *ninety-two* afflictions that the FDA itself has listed as possibly related to aspartame use: blindness, comas, weakness, memory loss, anxiety, cramps, joint pain, insomnia, spasms, rashes, palpitations, diarrhea, fatigue, numbness, irritability, dizziness, fainting, panic, weight gain, depression, nausea, headaches, loss of diabetic control, burning tongue, loss of taste, chest pain, tinnitus, deafness, slurred speech, and four different types of seizures. Years ago the FDA had already listed ten thousand consumer aspartame complaints.

More than sixty million dollars worth of diet cola was dumped in Europe several years ago because people in three nations reported nausea, headaches, and other symptoms after drinking it. There are even those who suspect that the so-called "Gulf War syndrome" may have been triggered, at least in part, by truckloads of diet soda that sat in the Arabian sun for months before being consumed. A 1993 study showed aspartame is mutagenic, causing mutations and birth defects, one of the main symptoms associated with those who claim to have been poisoned by *something* during the Gulf War.

Aspartame Seems to Target the Brain.

Aspartame has been shown to have great impact on many of the chemical reactions in the brain. It negatively effects dopamine, cerebral cholecystokinin (CCK), serotonin, endorphins, other important neurotransmitters, the permeability of the blood-brain barrier to phenylalanine, and insulin.

Too much aspartic acid, a component of Aspartame kills certain neurons in the brain by allowing the influx of too much calcium into the cells. This influx, in turn, triggers excessive amounts of free radicals, which stimulate or "excite" the neural cells to death.

Dr. Olney confirmed for me that holes in the brain have been directly linked to the consumption of aspartic acid (aspartame) in research studies involving laboratory animals. According to Dr. Russell Blaylock the same results occur with consumption of glutamic acid (MSG).

In inhibiting the production of serotonin, aspartame causes mood swings and a *craving for carbohydrates*. In my office, I have discovered in talking with my clients that those who drink diet sodas tend to eat more sweets and carbohydrates than those who don't. A product intended to help with *dieting* actually seems to promote *eating foods that cause you to become fat!*

Can we say definitively that aspartame *causes* brain cancer in human beings? No. The reason is that in order to prove such a relationship, a person would have to be given aspartame with the intent of trying to induce brain cancer. Nobody in their right mind would agree to such a study and no ethical researcher would ever ask that such a study be undertaken. We cannot say, therefore, that from a purely scientific standpoint aspartame causes brain cancer, but I *believe* that there is a cause-and-effect relationship. The evidence coming from animal studies is too compelling.

"Well, those findings are with rats," you may be saying. It's actually very difficult to cause spontaneous brain tumors in laboratory animals. Most substances that are tested on lab rats generate a result of .6 percent—that's less than one percent. When Dr. John Olney fed aspartame to rats in a pre-approval study, he had a result of 3.75 percent![2] That's a significant study by any scientific accounts and it should have signaled sufficient cause for more study of the chemical. It didn't.

Cellular Phones or Aspartame?

We have all heard media reports not too long ago that the use of cellular phones may be linked to brain cancer. One of the underlying factors that led to these reports was the documentation of a major increase in brain cancer in our nation. Researchers began to scramble for clues as to why this dramatic increase was occurring.

What the cellular phone critics could not explain, however, is why the increase in brain cancer has been approximately the same for adults and *children*. Three-year-olds are not frequent cell-phone users! What we do know with documentation is that diet soft drinks and other so-called diet foods using aspartame are consumed by adults and children in nearly identical percentages. Furthermore, Dr. Olney's study indicates that pregnant women who consume aspartame during their pregnancy are highly correlative with their children who develop brain cancer. There is also a high correlation between brain cancer development and elderly people with suppressed immune systems who consume large amounts of aspartame. This is probably what happened to my friend Howard.

Before we leave the cellular phone issue entirely, let me quickly note that the microwave radiation used in cellular phone technology is very powerful. I am not completely dismissing the potential for a relationship between frequent cellular phone use and brain cancer.

What I am saying is that the correlation between aspartame and brain cancer is far more likely! Remember, I have already warned you to stay away from microwaves that are in use. Now I am warning you to use a hands-free set if you use a cellular phone.

Aspartame is Highly Addictive.

Some of the withdrawal effects noted in various research studies have been fairly violent and often prolonged. The anecdotal evidence associated with these withdrawal effects is mountain-high and it isn't fun to read. Most of the people who admit they are aspartame addicts continually refer to the terrible way they feel if they try to wean themselves off aspartame; nearly all consider it nearly impossible to stop using aspartame.

The symptoms are not only physical, but mental. Severe confusion and memory loss has been noted, as well as depression and suicidal tendencies. Those who are addicted to aspartame and who were formally addicted to alcohol or amphetamines have said repeatedly that stopping aspartame use is *much* more difficult than stopping their drinking or pill-popping. I have a dear pastor friend who is so addicted to aspartame that he cannot stop drinking diet sodas, regardless of how much information I give him about aspartame and how much he *admits* to wanting to stop. I find this both troubling and sad.

What many are starting to recognize is that aspartame-based sodas first quench thirst, and then *cause* thirst. The more you drink aspartame-laced sodas, the more you desire them.

The addictive power of aspartame seems especially potent in children. Those who are denied aspartame sodas after drinking them regularly tend to manifest extreme hyperactivity and aggressive behaviors. More information on some childhood behavioral problems can be found in my *Eat, Drink and Be Healthy* audio tape series.

You may be asking yourself, why aspartame is still on the market. Profit has got to be what keeps this toxin on the market, plus a national addiction to it. Thousands of companies use it in their products, which translates to billions of dollars in sales worldwide.

"But, Ted," you may be saying, "isn't aspartame FDA-approved?"

Are you aware that 50 percent of the drugs that are approved by the FDA are pulled from the market within five years after their release for public consumption, or are ordered to significantly alter their warning labeling to indicate additional side effects? Concerns and questions about aspartame have been raised by the Public Board of Inquiry (PBI) and FDA scientists, but approval has not been withdrawn. Just because a product bears FDA approval does not mean it is *safe* for you to consume! Other factors may be at work.

Furthermore, once a product has been approved by the FDA it is very difficult to have that action reversed. Financial and political forces become involved.

Researchers at the Massachusetts Institute of Technology (MIT) surveyed eighty people who suffered brain seizures after eating or drinking products with aspartame. Their report said, "These eighty cases meet the FDA's own definition of an imminent hazard to the public health, which requires the FDA to expeditiously remove a product from the market." The FDA has failed to act.

The National Soft Drink Association issued a thirty-page protest questioning the safety of aspartame in 1983. The soft drink manufacturers ignored it.

Dr. H. J. Roberts, a world expert on diabetes, listed fifty-eight diabetic aspartame reactions in a 1987 abstract and has said, "I now advise all patients with diabetes and hypoglycemia to avoid aspartame products." The American Diabetic Association ignored his work.

I cannot overemphasize my conclusion about aspartame: *Do not use it!* In my opinion, this is the most dangerous product ever to be released for general consumption into the population. If you need more information and research to convince you about aspartame, please see my book *Maximum Energy.*

What about Saccharin?

Saccharin is also an artificial, low-calorie sweetener often found in restaurants and other outlets. Is it safe? Some studies have shown saccharin to have harmful effects when fed to laboratory rats, but these effects pale in comparison to the magnitude or severity of the effects associated with aspartame. If you absolutely *must* reach for an artificial sweetener, I suggest you reach for a pink packet instead of a blue one.

STEVIA—THE NATURAL SWEETENER

Stevia stands in sharp contrast to aspartame. Stevia has not made the big time on the sweetener scene, probably because it doesn't hold huge potential for a chemical company patent. But stevia is far sweeter than sugar, can be used in baking and cooking (unlike aspartame), is safe for diabetics, and is calorie-free.

As far as I am concerned, stevia offers an ideal alternative to sugars and sugar substitutes. It is the ideal sweetener for anyone who is obese or who suffers from diabetes, hypoglycemia, high blood pressure, or chronic yeast infections. It has all the benefits of artificial sweeteners and none of the drawbacks.

Stevia, known officially as *Stevia rebaudianada,* is also called *sweet herb* or *honey leaf.* It comes from the leaves of a shrub that belongs to the aster or chrysanthemum family of plants. It is found primarily in the Paraguayan mountains, but more than two hundred species of stevia have been identified around the world. A fine white powder can be extracted from the leaves of the plant and this common form of the herb is known as stevioside.

Stevia has been rated as from fifty to four hundred times sweeter than white sugar but it does not adversely effect blood sugar levels and is nontoxic. It inhibits the formation of cavities and plaque. It contains no artificial ingredients. It has not been linked to microorganisms such as bacteria or yeast.

Because stevia is so sweet, the most frequent mistake people make with the powdered stevia is using too much. Very tiny amounts of the powder can have a powerful effect. In fact, liquid extracts should be measured in drops. One half to one teaspoon of the liquid achieves the same effect as one cup of white sugar. If the powdered form is used, it should be mixed with hot water to create a more workable concentrate. Hot liquids seem to release the sweetening power of stevia more rapidly. This concentrate can then be refrigerated and measured out with an eye dropper.

Stevia works particularly well with dairy products (sweetening non-fat yogurt, for example), fruit dishes, beverages, and fresh desserts. It can be combined with molasses, honey, maple syrup, and fructose to maximize their sweetness, and thus minimize their use. It does not work well with yeast breads, which require sugar to rise. Baking with stevia is best if the recipes have a distinct flavor such as lemon or cinnamon. Baked goods sweetened with stevia do not brown as much as those baked with sugar.

In various countries around the world, stevia has been used for hundreds of years without any recorded side effects. No anomalies have ever been observed in cell, enzyme, chromosomal or other significant physiological functions. It has never been associated with any forms of cancer or birth defects.

The Japanese especially have studied stevia. One study conducted in 1987 concluded that more than 170 metric tons of stevia had been consumed in Japan in 1987, with no documented side effects.[4]

Clinical studies have shown that stevia actually increases glucose tolerance and decreases blood sugar levels. It has also been used as a digestive aid for many years in areas where the plant grows freely. It is not only a do-no-harm sweetener, but it actually is a helpful herb for the body!

Some people who have used stevia have found that their hunger decreases dramatically if they take stevia drops fifteen to twenty minutes before a meal. While there are no scientific studies to measure this effect, experts have presumed that the glycosides in stevia help to reset the appetite mechanism in the brain, providing a feeling of satisfaction.

You will find stevia in your health food store, sold as a "dietary supplement" rather than a sweetening agent. Like many herbs, it has a topical use as well as an oral use—it has been used for years in South American to heal wounds. Some have also used it to soften and tone the skin and to ease wrinkles and lines. (Liquid extracts can be applied directly to the skin.)

DIET PILLS AND CANDIES

The only actual drug approved by the U.S. Food and Drug Administration for weight-loss purposes is phenylpropanolamine (PPA), which is sold under trade names such as Dexatrim and Acutrim. If that chemical name sounds a lot like an amphetamine, you should know that PPA is structurally similar to amphetamines, which were the original diet pills. PPA also acts as a decongestant and is found in cold medications such as Contact and Dristan. In fact, it's an ingredient in more than one hundred medications. Americans annually take sixteen billion doses of PPA—four billion doses are in the form of diet pills.

Although PPA has been around since 1939, and fairly heavily marketed to the public since the 1960s, it is only in the 1980s that studies began to question PPA's appetite-suppressing ability. One study found that its actual weight-loss effects are meager—patients in one trial who took PPA over a six-week period lost only two pounds more than a placebo control group. A 1983 study found that PPA can cause blood pressure problems when combined with caffeine, a common mixture until 1983. PPA has also been linked to strokes.

Most over-the-counter diet aids are actually a combination of various vitamins, minerals, herbs, and fiber.

The people who take them rarely understand, however, what they are taking and what the possible effects may be in their bodies.

OVER-THE-COUNTER WEIGHT-LOSS FORMULAS

If you choose to take any over-the-counter or specialty weight-loss enhancing formulas, be sure to:

- read the labels carefully. Know what you are putting into your body!

- follow recommended dosages carefully. Do not overdose or self-prescribe your use of these products.

- take the products according to package directions. Some products recommend the tablets be taken on an empty stomach, some on a full stomach, some at breakfast time, and others later in the day.

- read any of the contraindications and take them seriously. Know what the potential side effects may be.

- make sure it doesn't contain aspartame.

Let me warn you in advance. Every product carries with it certain warnings and precautions, but you may need to pull out a magnifying glass to read them. Some manufacturers put this information only on the packaging box, not on the bottle inside the box. Make the effort to read what you are putting into your system. The manufacturers are definitely trying to prevent you from reading the warning labels and finding out the truth about their product.

Especially heed those warnings that refer to pregnant or lactating women, persons under the age of eighteen, and those with high blood pressure, epilepsy, glaucoma, thyroid or heart disease, or any other specific ailments that may be identified.

Also be aware that many of these products have interactions when they are combined with other medications, especially cough, cold and allergy medications, decongestants, MAO inhibitors, antidepressants, and even caffeine.

Since I do not like these over-the-counter diet products, I never recommend them. If you are determined to take them, however, I do not recommend that you exceed the recommended dose per day.

If you find your sleep disrupted, you are taking too much. If you experience tremors, nervousness, heart palpitations, or tingling sensations, stop taking the product.

Some products are packaged as candy, tea, or beverage drinks. Don't assume that you can use them as freely as you might pop M&Ms or drink water. Not so! These are powerful medicines—treat them as such.

Do not use these products if you are more than 20 percent over your desired weight without seeking professional advice from your physician.

Keep in mind always that most of these products have a statement associated with them that reads something like this: "For best results, use as part of a low-fat diet and exercise program." The fact is, if you really are following a good eating and exercise program, you likely won't need the product at all!

Furthermore, these products often make the disclaimer, "For temporary or short-term weight loss." These products are not for the long haul of maintaining fat loss. For that, you are going to have to exercise and eat properly for the rest of your life.

HOW LIGHT IS "LIGHT"?

Watch out for the word "light" on packaging labels! A number of so-called diet products are on the market using the words "light," "low-calorie," "fewer calories," and "reduced calories." These terms can be very deceptive since they can be used to describe any food that has reduced fat by 50 percent or calories by 33 percent. This does not mean that the product is ultimately low fat.

The term *reduced fat* can also be deceiving. Low-fat or reduced-fat foods must have 25 percent less fat than the same brand's regular counterpart. Let me give you an example. One super-premium ice cream normally has sixteen grams of fat per half cup. A version of the same ice cream with only twelve grams per half cup is labeled "reduced fat"! That's high-fat consumption any way you label it.

Also be aware that some products have cut fat but increased sugar. In one fig-bar product, the fat-free bar has almost four teaspoons of sugar per serving. That's still a high-calorie bar! In fact, that particular bar has one hundred calories while the regular version has one hundred and ten calories. Not much difference and remember that sugar spikes your blood sugar quickly and then is stored as fat.

It's actually a fairly widespread practice for companies to use more sugar in the products that have fat eliminated. Sugar is used to create a better taste and texture. Nearly all manufacturers ADD sugar when they take away fat.

When comparing products, always make sure you

- evaluate equal serving sizes.

- compare sodium amounts.

- compare calories.

- compare the number of fat grams.

- compare the number of sugar grams.

Be sure to note any disclaimers at the end of the fat-free ingredients. A product may have up to .5 gram of fat per serving and still legally claim to be fat-free.

THINK FRESH, NOT PACKAGED

If you truly want "diet" food, go the produce section of your grocery store. Nature has already produced the very best diet foods in the form of fruit and fresh green and yellow vegetables. Choose *organic* produce. Choose *ripe* produce. Choose *beautiful* produce. And enjoy the taste without any chemical aftertaste!

Not only will these fruits and vegetables provide healthful nutrients rather than harmful chemicals, they will give you important fiber. And that's where we turn next.

KEY #8:

Take in sufficient fiber every day.

14

FIBER—THE KEY TO TRANSPORTING FAT OUT OF YOUR BODY

When I do my live seminars, I often ask the crowd for a show of hands concerning various topics I'm discussing. I never ask, however, for a show of hands when it comes to constipation. I know, however, that in any audience I address, at least half of the people there have this problem either chronically or periodically. That's the statistical norm for the adult population of our nation. A recognized authority on colon hygiene, V. E. Irons has stated that the U.S. Public Health Service estimates that 90 percent of all Americans have a clogged colon to some degree![1]

The solution to most constipation problems—one without side effects—may be as simple as dietary fiber.

Most Americans do not get enough dietary fiber in the foods they eat day by day. The human digestive system, and particularly the large intestine and colon, become impacted when too little dietary fiber and water are consumed.

Constipation and the Obese

Constipation seems especially to be a problem for those who are obese.

Several years ago I read an article in which a medical examiner autopsied the body of an obese man and found that his colon weighed sixty pounds! The colon is an elastic organ that expands and opens up to incredible proportions when necessary. Some people who have been autopsied have had colons measuring nine inches in diameter (the colon is normally two inches in diameter). A great deal of weight can be kept in the colon of the body. The best way to get rid of that weight in a hurry is to increase your dietary fiber and drink sufficient water.

How Much Fiber?

You need to be eating between twenty-five and thirty grams of fiber *daily*. Many of my clients admit to me that they have trouble consuming thirty grams of fiber a *week*.

Most of the foods Americans seem to love to eat, such as pasta, breads, meats, dairy products, and virtually all junk food, have little or no fiber at all. One serving of bran flakes has about four grams of fiber and a large unpeeled apple has between three and four grams of fiber.

To make sure you get twenty to thirty grams of fiber, you must have fiber at breakfast and at least five servings of low-glycemic fresh fruit and vegetables daily. (That's also the number of servings recommended by the American Cancer Society.)

GOOD SOURCES OF FIBER

Fiber is the part of your food that your digestive system cannot digest. Your parents probably called it *roughage* or *bulk*. Dietary fiber is most abundant in plant products such as fruits, grains, and vegetables. It is also commonly associated with bran, the outer husk of most grains.

There are two forms of fiber: soluble and insoluble. Soluble fiber dissolves easily in water. It is absorbed in the intestine and circulated in the bloodstream. Soluble fiber in the blood has a great advantage in fat loss since the fiber attaches itself to blood fats and creates a complex that removes these fats from the blood system. The net result for most people is not only the elimination of fat from the body, but a lowering of cholesterol.[2]

Insoluble fiber absorbs water, also, but it is not absorbed in the intestine. It remains there to form a bulk mass that serves to sweep bodily wastes through the intestines, large intestine, and colon, and out of the body. Without sufficient fiber, food wastes, including disease-causing toxins, move slowly through the colon, if at all. This mass can then putrefy right in the body. The result is not only constipation, but the release of toxic materials into the bloodstream.

Fiber includes cellulose, hemicellulose, lignins, pectins, gums, mucilages, and storage polysaccharides. The majority of plant fibers (the first three listed above) are insoluble. Pectin, found in fruits, is soluble.

Fiber is also commonly associated with bran, the outer husk of most grains. It is very important that when you choose grains, you choose the bulkiest grains possible—ones that still have the bran included. Look for whole bran, whole wheat, and other whole-grain products.

Fiber Supplements

I also recommend to my clients that they take a fiber supplement several times a week. I use coarse wheat bran, oat bran, or psyllium on a regular basis. Oat bran has been shown in research studies to be superior to wheat and corn bran in its ability to lower blood fats.[3]

Psyllium husks are pure fiber. This product is generally sold in bulk and is taken in a dosage of one tablespoon about a half hour before a meal with a large glass of water. Drink the mixture quickly. Psyllium husks give a full feeling and cut down any hunger pangs you may feel on a fat-loss program. This form of fiber seems especially good for those with high or low blood sugar problems.

Glucomannan is another good fiber product. It is derived from the edible root of the konjac plant (*Amorphollaus konjac*), which is in the same family as the yam. The Japanese have used this plant for centuries for fiber in their diet. This product works primarily by gently swelling the stomach, bringing a feeling of fullness. Glucomannan expands fifty to sixty times in size when it reaches the stomach. The recommended dose is one thousand milligrams, which usually means taking two five hundred-milligram capsules or tablets. The product should be taken with eight ounces of water a half hour before a meal.

Some people can feel a bit bloated when they begin to use glucomannan. If that happens, cut the dose in half for two or three days to let your system adjust. In most health food stores, you'll find this product available in powder, capsule, cake, tablet, cookie, and candy forms.

When Taking Supplemental Fiber

Always take supplemental fiber separately from other supplements and medications. You don't want to bind and flush valuable nutrients or medications from your system before they have a chance to enter your bloodstream.

If you are purchasing a fiber supplement, look for pectin and various fruit fibers on the label. Make sure you chew any crackers or wafers very well and that you drink at least eight ounces of water with them—the same amount of water as if you are taking fiber tablets.

As mentioned before, fiber is best taken a half hour before a meal so the stomach has an opportunity to register a fuller feeling before you eat. You may experience a bit of stomach growling if you are not accustomed to having fiber in your system. If this happens, reduce the amount you are taking for two or three days and then gradually increase the dosage.

When using fiber products—tablets or bulk—be sure you take supplemental vitamins and minerals since large amounts of fiber can interfere with the absorption of nutrients from the food you eat. Again, if possible with the exception of my protein shake recipe do not take these supplements *with* the fiber—take them at other times of the day.

THE IMPORTANCE OF STAYING REGULAR

I once had a client say to me that she was very regular. To her, regularity meant a regular bowel movement one day a week. She was anything but regular! Another client, whose health was a wreck, admitted she had a bowel movement only once a month. That's like only throwing out the garbage from your house once a month. Bodily waste needs to be eliminated *daily*—ideally two or three times a day.

What about over-the-counter chemical laxatives? I discourage their use. They may help you eliminate bodily waste but these laxatives are very harsh on the system and are habit forming. Bulk laxatives, by comparison are not chemical products. They simply provide the fiber needed to form a bowel movement.[4]

Not only does sufficient dietary fiber help in the removal of fat globules from the bloodstream, it also can reduce atherosclerosis (hardening of the arteries). An increase in dietary fiber is the mainstay treatment for hemorrhoids.[5] Fiber also offers protection from cancer of the colon, prostate, and breast.

High-fiber diets have been proven to be helpful in the control of blood sugar levels in diabetics, especially those having Type II diabetes. Some researchers have suggested that a high-fiber diet can actually lead to such great improvement for Type II diabetics that they are able to decrease or eliminate their need for diabetic medications.[6]

In another study, those who followed an eating plan that added one hundred grams of dietary fiber to their diet each week experienced a reduction in their blood pressure.[7] The subjects in yet another study showed an average 10 percent drop in their blood pressure readings after only two weeks on a high-fiber diet.[8]

CLEANSING YOUR SYSTEM

Fiber is an ongoing help to the person who is pursuing a fat-loss program. Sometimes an initial cleansing of the digestive tract is beneficial to rid the body of toxins and help restore colon function to a normal state. There are two main ways to jump-start this cleansing process in order to get maximum benefit not only from fiber, but from all nutrients you take into your system.

Colonic Cleansing

A number of my clients have benefited from a colonic cleansing program. Many physicians have chosen to prescribe synthetic laxatives to their patients rather than suggest this procedure. A colonic cleansing program cleanses the *entire length* of the colon, compared to only about twelve inches of the colon for an enema. A thoroughly cleansed colon can be a good way to start a fat-loss program. Immediately after such a cleansing, a person needs to make sure that he or she has adequate daily fiber and water to keep the colon cleansed from toxic build-up. Colonic cleansing should not be over-used or used as a substitute for taking fiber. (If you want more information about colonic cleansing programs, give my office a call at 1-800-726–1834.)[9]

Fasting

Fasting has some advantages in weight loss, but be cautious. Long periods of fasting or frequent fasting are not advisable! The advantages of a short fast—not more than a few days—can be these:

- The digestive tract has a chance to totally cleanse itself of accumulated waste and putrefactive bacteria.

- Generally speaking, the universal solvent—water—is consumed in large volume on a fast. This can help to purify the kidneys and bloodstream in a way that is impossible when a person is eating regularly.

- A mental clarity is achieved during a fast, which can be beneficial in helping you refocus your goals and priorities regarding your health. It's often amazing how clear a person's thinking can become when chemicals and food additives are removed from the bloodstream—and especially how clear the thinking becomes regarding health matters! A fast can give a psychological jump-start to a fat-loss plan.

- The stomach has a chance to shrink back in size, which can make it easier for a person to control the quantity of food that is consumed.

- Fasting also heightens the senses, including the sense of taste. You will likely find that you have a new appreciation for the taste of food after a short fast.

- A fast provides an intermission, of sorts, in your life habits. It's easier to establish new habits after breaking with the old.

A three-day fast is usually sufficient. Prolonged fasting burns up muscle tissue as well as fat. That is why when clients start on a seven day cleansing program, I provide them with concentrated nutrients to help prevent protein catabolism. Also, I feel that you should never fast for more than one day without the use of colonics, which by the way can be done at home. Never fast for longer than seven days in a row without being under the care of a physician.[9]

During the fast drink only vegetable juices or clear low-sodium broths and bouillons. The juice should be fresh, not canned—ideally juices should be ones you make yourself in a juicer. Pure freshly squeezed beet juice is considered the best fasting juice. Be sure to drink lots of distilled water with lemon juice throughout each day—even more than half your weight in ounces.

As you end your fast, limit your eating the next day to two protein drinks (morning and afternoon; you can divide them among four mini-meals) and eat steamed, watery vegetables and take dietary fiber tablets (or psyllium).

THE BASICS

Thus far we have covered six basic tips that relate to what you take into your body on a fat-loss program:

1. Eat six meals a day.

2. Eat protein at every meal.

3. Eat low-glycemic-index carbohydrates.

4. Eliminate all foods that are bad for you.

5. Drink half your weight in ounces of pure water a day.

6. Take in sufficient fiber.

There's one more key to *eating* on a fat-loss diet and its the one you probably think least likely: Eat fat. You need some at every meal, but only specific kinds. That's next.

KEY #9:

**Eat "essential" fatty acids
at every meal.**

15

NOT ALL FATS ARE BAD—
SOME ARE *ESSENTIAL*

Twenty-five years ago, most people—even nutritional scientists—lumped all fats together into one giant, greasy lump. Now, however, we have become fat savvy and we know that some fats are actually good for a person, and especially helpful in a fat-loss plan.

There are three basic rules related to your eating of fat:

1. Never eat a fat-free meal. Some fat needs to be taken along with your protein and carbohydrates at every meal.

2. Limit your total intake of fat each day. Be sure to keep your fat intake at about 20 percent of your total daily calories. Brett Hall, R.D., who is a director of research and development for experimental and applied sciences, has said,

> Despite popular belief, it is not true that eliminating fat from your diet altogether will automatically make you lean. Your body needs some fat to stay healthy. Numerous studies have concluded that those who are most successful in losing fat and maintaining the loss are those who take in less than forty grams a day of fat in their diets.[1]

3. Eat the right kinds of fat. The right fats to eat are the main subject of this chapter.

THE RIGHT KINDS OF FAT . . . AND THE WRONG ONES!

I'm not going to try to give you a biochemistry course on fat, but there are a few facts about fats that you should know. From my point of view, the more you know about how your body works and why, the more you will want to choose those things that work well for your body and avoid those things that are harmful to it.

Fats fall into two groups: saturated and unsaturated.

Saturated Fats

Saturated fats are the ones usually found in meat and dairy products. The body uses them primarily for energy but not much else. What isn't used for energy goes into storage (usually into fat cells).

You'll especially want to steer clear of these three types of saturated fatty acids:

Stearic Acid This makes platelets in the blood stickier and more likely to form clots in blood vessels. Such clots increase the risk of stroke and heart attack. Stearic acid is found in high quantities in beef, mutton, and pork.

Palmitic Acid This is found in coconut and palm kernel oils.

Trans-Fats The most harmful fats of all are the trans-fats. These are usually labeled hydrogenated and partially hydrogenated. They are artificially processed and often mislabeled as polyunsaturated fats. They are the worst fats when it comes to heart disease and they have also been linked to breast cancer. They are *worse* for your cardiovascular system than saturated fats. Yes, margarine (a hydrogenated fat) is worse than the butyric acid in butter. Trans-fatty acids can cause a very rapid rise in cholesterol and triglyceride levels.

Hydrogenation, which basically is a process that exposes fats to the action of hydrogen, rearranges the molecular bonds on fatty acids. This process reduces the essential fatty acid content of both Omega-6 and Omega-3 oils. It causes trans-fatty acids (also called T-acids) to take the place of essential fatty acids in cell membranes, interfering with their metabolism and usurping some of the enzymes that produce important hormonelike substances called eicosanoids which are involved in many aspects of bodily functions. In laymen's terms this translates to mean that hydrogenated or partially hydrogenated fats are terrible for your health and will increase your risk of cancer and heart disease. Be sure to read your food labels!

Unsaturated Fats

Unsaturated fats generally come from plant products. The body uses these fats to construct cell membranes, support nerve function, and produce hormones. These fats can be used for energy if all these more vital needs have been met.

A certain amount of unsaturated fat is needed just to survive. Two particular types of fat are essential for health. They are known as Omega-6 fatty acids and Omega-3 fatty acids. Together, the two types are known as *essential fatty acids* (EFA).

The body is capable of making many different kinds of fats, but it cannot make Omega-6 or Omega-3. They have to be supplied through the diet. Hence the term *essential.*

Regardless of the type of fat, each produces nine calories of energy per gram, although your body prefers to save essential fatty acids for hormonelike functions rather than burn them for energy. These fats actually stimulate metabolism and speed up the rate the body burns fat and glucose. In other words, eating essential fatty acids actually helps the body burn up fat.

You may not find Omega-6 and Omega-3 on a label. The more common names for these fats are *linoleic* and *linolenic.*

These two terms are so similar that I'm going to emphasize their difference in the next few paragraphs. LinoLEic fat is found in most vegetable oils—which are nearly always highly processed and filled with free radicals and trans-fatty acids. While linoLEic fatty acids are good, the bad of the trans-fats outweighs their good in these oils, and especially so when the oils are heated for cooking purposes.

Trans-fatty acids can contribute to heart disease, lower immunity, decrease testosterone, and damaged insulin responsiveness, and add to the size and number of fat cells in the body.

A good source of linoLEic acid is evening primrose oil. Evening primrose oil has been shown to be highly effective in lowering blood pressure, normalizing fat metabolism in diabetics, preventing liver damage, helping with fat loss, and even improving the condition of a person's hair and nails.[2]

LinoLENic acid, the second essential fatty acid, is found in soy, walnut, and hemp oils, and in dark-green vegetable leaves. You'd have to eat a whole lot of those leaves, however, to get enough. Flax oil is the richest source of linoLENic acid.

You can find both linoLEic and linoLENic fatty acids in a supplement called gamma-linolenic acid (GLA). Recommended dosage is 250 international units (IU) a day—there is no known toxicity level. GLA is formed from the active ingredients in borage oil, black currant seed oil, flaxseed oil, and evening primrose oil.

There's yet another bit of chemistry that's good to know. Two of the essential fatty acids have the nearly impossible to pronounce names of docosahexaenoic acid and eicosapentaenoic acid. DHA and EPA for short. These oils have been shown to lower blood pressure, improve cholesterol, prevent cancer, and improve the general balance of the bloodstream. They have profound hormonal effects.[3] Fish oils are the most valuable source of DHA and EPA.

What Essential Fatty Acids Do for Your Body.

Essential fatty acids (EFA) are required for the transport and metabolism of both cholesterol and triglycerides. An eating plan with sufficient EFAs has been shown to lower high cholesterol levels by up to 25 percent and high triglyceride levels by up to 65 percent.

Essential fatty acids are also required for the normal development of the brain. In adults, they are required for good brain function. In the human fetus, the brain begins to develop six weeks after conception and that development continues until one year after birth. It is vitally important that pregnant and lactating women have sufficient fatty acids in their eating program.

Essential fatty acids are related to various specific cellular functions. They stimulate metabolism, increase the metabolic rate, increase oxygen uptake, and increase energy production. And finally, essential fatty acids slow the growth of cancer cells.

These fatty acids function in the body to regulate platelet stickiness, arterial muscle tone, inflammatory responses, sodium excretion through the kidneys, and immune functions, and to stimulate immune responses.

The essential fatty acids have a profound effect on the nervous system as well. As an interesting side note, hyperactive and attention-deficit children have shown remarkable improvements in health, stamina, and concentration when given increased amounts of essential fatty acids. Severe thirst, which is a significant symptom in hyperactive children, is a cardinal sign of a deficiency of essential fatty acids.

All of which is to say, fatty acids are *essential.* You must have an adequate amount of them daily—not only for your fat-loss program but for your overall health, not only now but for the rest of your life.[4]

Function of Prostaglandins

Let's assume for a minute that your body is getting the proper amounts and types of both linoleic and linolenic acids. What happens then? Well, in an ideal biochemical state, these oils make other fatty acids, which impact the function of Prostaglandins (PGs). These are the real keys to controlling your body's metabolism.

PGs made from linoLEic acid have a host of beneficial effects: They relax blood vessels, improve circulation, lower blood pressure, decrease inflammation, improve nerve function, regulate calcium metabolism, improve T-cell function, and prevent release of harmful arachidonic acid from cells.

PGs made from linoLENic acid also prevent degenerative cardio-vascular changes.

All of which is to conclude: You *want* an adequate amount of fatty acids working for you at all times.

AN EASY WAY TO TAKE ESSENTIAL FATTY ACIDS

How can you go about getting a sufficient quantity of the right kinds of fat in your system? First, you can include foods in your eating plan that are high in these fatty acids: Avocados, olives, raw nuts and seeds, and wheat and corn germ are sources of good fats that contain essential fatty acids. Do not, however, make these foods the mainstay of your eating plan. Use them in moderation—no more than twice a week.

These are other foods high in essential fatty acids:

- Flax oil and walnuts are high in ALA. (While flax seed oil is good for ALA, it also slows down the fat burning metabolism.)
- Cod liver oil and cold water fish are good sources of EPA.
- Algae derived supplements, cod liver oil, and cold water fish provide DHA.
- Evening primrose oil, borage oil, and black currant seed oil are sources for GLA. (These oils help stimulate the fat burning metabolism.)

The Easy Supplemental Way

But let me make it even easier for you! You can get all of the essential fatty acids you need each day by taking three supplements:

- 1,200 milligrams of Borage oil (a rich source of linolenic acid)

- 1,200 milligrams of fish oil (cod liver oil, for DHA and EPA)

- 600 milligrams of evening primrose oil (for GLA)

Look for borage oil in two-hundred-IU capsules (one per meal), cod liver oil in two hundred IU capsules (six per meal), and evening primrose oil in one hundred IU capsules (one per meal).

Eight capsules of oil per meal. What could be easier?

"But, Ted," you may be arguing, "I remember cod liver oil from my childhood. Yech!"

The capsules of cod liver oil have no taste. You'll find, however, that the liquid is less expensive and works much faster so if you can handle the taste, I recommend the liquid form.

A word about flaxseed oil. It should not be taken in quantities greater than 1,200 milligrams a day. However, on a fat-loss program, larger quantities are excellent for immune system support.

The Great Benefits of Cod Liver Oil

I am a strong advocate for cod liver oil. In fact, if you only take *one* fatty-acid product, I recommend that it be at least six capsules of cod-liver oil per meal. Why? Because cod liver oil aids a number of biochemical functions and slows the absorption of calories into the body. This, in turn, helps a person to feel full longer and reduces the Syndrome X associated with an insulin release into the body.

Let me briefly remind you of some of the information we covered earlier in this book about how insulin works in the body. Its function is similar to that of a thermostat. When the temperature in a house hits the predetermined temperature level set on the thermostat, the air conditioning or heating system is triggered. When the body's blood glucose level moves past a certain point, the pancreas "turns on" and releases insulin into the system to reduce the glucose level to what is normal for the body.

Insulin functions as a storage hormone for the extra glucose, which the body stores as fat. Insulin doesn't care where the extra calories come from initially—fat, carbohydrates, or protein. Any extra calories that aren't used are stored as fat.

Why, then, should we make careful food choices? Sugar-based foods are high glycemic—which means that they break down very quickly into glucose and give a major rush of glucose into the system. They spike the system with glucose. This spike is then matched by a spike of insulin release and the excess glucose is stored as fat, even before that glucose has an opportunity to feed or fuel important body cells. People who live off donuts, or even rice cakes or potatoes, are ingesting almost pure sugar into their systems. Potatoes turn to glucose in the bloodstream faster than table sugar! That's why the glycemic index is such an important tool for evaluating what we eat if our goal is maximum fat loss.

When different foods are combined, the resulting amount of glucose released into the body varies, so a simplistic reading of the glycemic index is not always valid. We can learn to avoid high-glycemic foods, however, and in a later chapter we will discuss this further. What is important for you to understand at this point is that *cod liver oil taken at each meal helps to regulate this glucose release into the blood stream and lowers the amount of fat-storing insulin that is simultaneously released.*

THE BEST OILS TO USE IN COOKING AND SALAD DRESSING

I recommend that you use olive oil in your cooking and salad dressings rather than any other kind of oil.

The healthiest oils are those that have less saturated fat and low ratios of Omega-6 to Omega-3. Olive oil is the best, followed by flaxseed oil and walnut oil.

And the worst oils? Coconut oil is the highest in saturated fat (around 78 percent!) It has no Omega-3 and less than two percent

Omega-6. Safflower, Crisco, and corn oils are all high in saturated fat and have poor ratios of Omega-6. Shortening, which is hydrogenated, is the worst choice!

FAT TO LOSE FAT

It seems ironic doesn't it that essential fatty acids can actually help you lose fat. Nevertheless, it's biochemically true. When people pursue a totally fat-free diet they get into serious trouble. You need some fat to keep your system humming and lubricated. Good fats do that. Bad fats just clog up the works.

Having covered the seven basics of eating on a fat-loss plan, we turn now to the right kinds of *exercise* to do on a fat-loss plan.

Put on your walking shoes!

What About Cholesterol?

I continue to meet people who think that cholesterol is fat, or that it is related to the fat content of food. Cholesterol actually has nothing to do with the fat content of a food. Cholesterol is a steroid produced by the liver. Only animal products contain it. A food item can have no cholesterol and yet be high in fat, and conversely, something high in cholesterol can be low in fat. However, a diet high in fat, particularly saturated fat, can *raise* cholesterol levels because of a process that is triggered in the liver by high-fat intake.

KEY #10:

Do cardiovascular (aerobic) exercise five times a week for twenty-five minutes in the morning before eating anything.

KEY #11:

Do strength-building (weight) exercises and flexibility (stretching) exercises three to five times a week.

16

KEEP MOVING!

DON'T FADE AWAY INTO FLAB

Once a person passes the physical age of twenty, he or she loses 6 to 7 percent of their total muscle mass every ten years unless that person does resistant exercises regularly. Regular exercise is the key to keeping yourself from "fading away" as you advance in age.

Between the ages of twenty and seventy, the average person loses approximately 30 percent of their muscle mass due to tissue atrophy! And the bad news is this: Most of what replaces that muscle mass is fat.

The good news is that a loss of lean muscle mass can be prevented or greatly reduced in most cases through consistent strength-building exercises, and through a wise diet and plenty of pure water.

THE GREAT BENEFITS OF EXERCISE

Exercise provides five very important benefits to the human body:

1. Exercise increases lean body tissue.

2. Exercise (strength-building) is the only way to reshape your genetically predisposed body type.

3. Exercise burns fat.

4. Exercise raises a person's metabolic rate.

5. Exercise increases the sensitivity of cells to insulin, which allows the pancreas to produce less insulin and not become over-taxed.

And if those aren't reasons enough . . .

Exercise causes the brain to release endorphin neuropeptides. Most people who are health conscious have heard about endorphin "highs"—the feeling of well-being after vigorous exercise. People who are physically fit can induce the release of these hormones more readily and in greater amounts. In other words, the more you train, the better you feel. But besides making you feel better, endorphins are also known to have beneficial effects on the immune system. Many white blood cells can bind to the neuropeptides.

Exercise also reduces the level of stress hormones, particularly the catecholamines. When these stress hormones are suppressed, immunity suffers.

Exercise is not just good for your muscles and your mind *today*, it's good for your *future* health and your ability to fight off the viruses and bacteria that may invade your body tomorrow.

THE THREE KINDS OF EXERCISE EVERYBODY NEEDS

The vast majority of Americans sit or lie down through most of their day. They lie down at night, of course, to sleep—that is about a third of one's day. Through the course of the day, most Americans sit behind the wheel of their cars, sit down at dinner tables, sit down at conference tables for meetings, sit down to watch television or roam the Internet, sit down while making telephone calls or having conversations with friends, and sit down at their desks to work. We have become a sedentary society and all the while, the fat has piled onto our bodies.

While I am writing about exercise, cardio, and lifting weights, it is crucial that you develop a burning desire to work out on a regular basis. Your workout has to become a priority in your life—not your main priority, but a priority none the less. So many people work out a few times and complain that they are sore, and after that their shadow never darkens the gym door again. Let me try to reframe how to look at being sore. If I work out and I don't get a little stiff or sore I don't feel as though my body received any benefit from the exercise. Being sore is not bad. It is what is supposed to happen after a good workout.

Let me give you just one example of dedication. It may seem a bit extreme to you but shows a can-do attitude regardless of the circumstances. Van Green, my NFL superstar friend, and I have known each other for over ten years. Van had been diligently working on becoming an ordained minister of the gospel and around seven years ago took a three-year hiatus from weight training.

Four years ago I was in need of a new workout partner. The gentleman I had been working out with was a well-known contractor in central Florida, and his business had grown so much it became necessary for him to adjust his workout schedule for a time that I couldn't train. So I called Van and asked him if he could arrange his schedule to work out with me early in the morning. His reply was an exuberant, "Yes!"

Van had really missed working out on a regular basis and was anxious to start back. Now remember, Van was 45 at the time, and I was 41. The first workout was a chest workout in which I took it real easy on Van because of his three-year layoff. The easy workout only frustrated Van. He was not sore at all. I had underestimated his incredible genetics. I mean, for all practical purposes, Van could play the role of Superman in the movie. Even today I joke with him after a hard workout and say, "Superman lives."

The next day, Van came in and said, "Don't take it easy on me. I am here to work out." What I heard him indirectly say was, don't waste my time again.

So I said to him, "Do you really want to go full-throttle on the leg workout today?"

His response was basically, "Give it your best shot." So I did.

Van stayed with me through an advance leg workout even after a three-year layoff. After the leg workout we did abdominals. (Most of you don't know that my second undergraduate degree from F.S.U. was in psychology and exercise physiology. That is why the exercise videos that I produce are so effective. Van and I did the advanced men's video workout. It is not for and should never be used by beginners. I have a beginning and intermediate men's videotape that is perfect for first timers and those who have been training for a year or so. (These tapes along with the women's exercise videos, are available through my office.)

Back to my story. Van was worn out and a little spacey after the workout I guess he figured that a white boy (Van and I joke about this all the time) couldn't put him through that intense of a workout. So I invited him to have a protein shake with me to help bring up his blood sugar. I told him to lie down on the back porch couch and relax and I would have his shake ready in a few minutes. (My wife has a rule: no stinky men in the house after a workout. Both Van and I needed a shower.)

Van said, "I will stay in the kitchen with you until the shake is done."

I replied, "You need to lie down. You haven't worked this hard in years." Before the words left my mouth, Van had passed out on my kitchen floor. Well, I knew this was a blood sugar related incident so I grabbed a pillow and put it under his head. By this time he was awake. He was laughing. I was laughing. My wife thought we were both nuts.

What had happened was that Van's blood sugar was so low that his brain was not getting sufficient glucose. Passing out was his body's only way to get him to lay down so that more blood and glucose could get to his brain. He was back to normal just a few minutes after drinking the protein shake.

The next day he was back for another workout and he has been with me ever since. That's dedication. That's commitment. That's a burning desire. That's consistency. That's character. That's not allowing circumstances to control your outcome. That's Van. And that's why I call him Superman.

I am in no way suggesting that you push yourself to this level of physical exhaustion. I am only relating this story because of its deeper meaning. Any exercise program should begin slowly until your body gets into shape. You will need to see your medical doctor first for a full physical before you begin any new exercise program.

If you are truly serious about maximum fat loss, you need to include three types of exercise in your weekly routine:

1. cardiovascular exercise (aerobics)

2. flexibility exercise (stretching)

3. strength-building exercise (weights)

Even if you haven't exercised regularly for years, you should start doing all three kinds of exercise. Set modest goals for yourself as you begin. Don't be reluctant to start out at a very simple, easy level.

CARDIOVASCULAR EXERCISE

You should be doing some kind of continuous cardiovascular exercise for twenty to thirty minutes at least three and preferably five times a week. Cardiovascular exercise is also called aerobics exercise, a phrase coined by Dr. Kenneth Cooper.

By cardiovascular exercise, I am referring to physical exertion that puts a healthy load on the heart, the lungs, and the complex network of blood vessels in your body (arteries, veins, and capillaries). Blood vessels and the heart are just like your muscles—they grow stronger with regular use and healthy exercise. The goal of cardiovascular exercise is to accelerate the heart rate for a sustained period of time and to burn body fat if needed.

If possible, engage in cardiovascular exercise first thing in the morning before any calories are eaten or drunk. (You may have water.) Exercising on an empty stomach causes the body to release glucagon from the pancreas to facilitate the burning of existing fat deposits for fuel. I personally lowered my own body fat levels by 5 percent in just one year by implementing this one change in my exercise program. On the other hand, if you eat something before you exercise, your body is going to use up only that food for energy. You won't be calling upon your body to draw on its fat reserves.

"Do I need to jog or run?" you may ask. No. In fact, I recommend *walking* for obese people and people over forty. It's much easier on the ligaments of the knees and hips.

"Only twenty to thirty minutes?" That's sufficient. Twenty minutes a day of walking on level ground has been shown to have very significant value in improving insulin sensitivity and glucose management.

Other than walking, the most popular cardiovascular exercises for the obese are swimming, cycling, low-impact aerobics, elliptical runners, and tread mills.

Don't try to accomplish your ultimate cardiovascular exercise goals the first day out! Bear in mind that you didn't get out of shape in a day and you aren't going to get back to a level of fitness in a day. If all you can do at the outset is to walk around the block every evening, then do it. If it's winter and too cold to walk where you live, get yourself a treadmill or an elliptical runner such as the Precor EFX544, which is what my wife and I use. If you can't walk fast enough at the outset to get your heart to a true cardiovascular workout rate, walk twenty minutes at the pace you *can* walk. Stay with your program and you will improve.

Adequately Warm Up

Always take time to warm up your muscles. Don't head out walking, cycling, or even swimming at full speed. Walk, cycle, or swim slowly for a few minutes to warm up your muscles, and then increase your speed for the bulk of your exercise time. Walk slowly for the last few minutes of your exercise session to give your muscles an opportunity to cool down.

There's an interesting word that the vast majority of people have never heard in relationship to their muscles: thixotropy. This word refers to the tendency of gels to be thick and viscous at rest, but pliant and fluid when they are shaken or otherwise disturbed. Although the thixotropic effect is not completely understood, scientists have speculated that after long periods of inactivity, muscle tissues begin to develop microscopic bonds, between both fibers and filaments. This phenomenon explains why we often feel stiff and creaky after getting up in the morning. It is also a reason that a warm-up session is important before active aerobic exercise. The warm-up raises the body temperature, which helps in muscle elongation, and helps to break down these bonds.

Later-in-the-Day Aerobics

One of the reasons many people give for not exercising daily is that they are "just too tired" or "too hungry" when they get home from work. I can understand both arguments. I'm generally tired and hungry when I get home from work too.

That's the reason that I strongly believe the best time to exercise is first thing in the morning before you have had anything to eat. If you try to schedule exercise into your day late in the day, too many things can crowd into that time. If you have a family waiting for you at home, it's difficult to stop by a gym after work. If you wait until after your evening meal to exercise, you'll find two dozen reasons not to put on those workout clothes. Try and get exercise out of the way first thing in the day. Remember, morning is the best time for burning fat.

If you must exercise later in the day, tell yourself that you'll actually be taking the edge off your hunger by exercising. Exercise shunts the blood away from the stomach and hunger pangs tend to disappear once you begin exercising. The good news, too, is that when you finish exercising, you'll actually be less hungry and want to eat less for your evening meal.

I once met a woman who swam in her apartment building's indoor pool every afternoon after work. The pool had a lifeguard, was heated year-round, and was located in the building's basement so it was readily accessible. She admitted to me, "I often went down to that pool exhausted from a hectic day and many times I thought to myself, *I just don't have the energy to swim this evening.* But then, I'd swim my twenty-four laps and discover when I went back in apartment that I had a new burst of energy for the evening. Plus I slept better when I actually did fall into bed at ten o'clock. When I didn't swim I found myself lethargic all evening and restless for at least an hour after I went to bed."

The real key, however, to feeling like exercise in the late afternoon or early evening is not to get overly hungry at any point during the day. Hunger is your body's natural signal that you need nutrients. By feeding your body six meals at regular intervals throughout a day, you will keep the edge off hunger at all times. "Needing food first" then becomes a moot argument.

Keeping Track of Your Progress

Keep a log of your cardiovascular workouts. Record the date, length of your exercise period, and the distance you cover. Also note any pain or discomfort that you felt when exercising. Note, too, any feelings you had while walking—perhaps a new awareness of something in the outdoors, a new appreciation for parts of your body, a new feeling of energy. Looking back on this log can give you a real sense of progress, and that, in turn, can motivate you to *maintain* your cardiovascular exercise. (An aerobics exercise log is provided for you in the *Maximum Fat Loss Workbook*.)

FLEXIBILITY EXERCISES

Flexibility is the ability to move muscles, joints, and bones with a full range of motion. Flexibility exercises are the way most of us achieve and maintain the maximum amount of flexibility we can enjoy. We used to call flexibility exercises *stretching exercises.*

Stretching is not only vital for flexibility, but in deterring joint and ligament problems. Flexibility exercises can greatly decrease the immobility that is so often associated with aging.

You should be doing a set of flexibility exercises at least three to four times a week, ideally after every morning cardiovascular workout.

I had back surgery in 1988 and during my recovery I implemented a daily stretching routine. It has made a huge difference in my flexibility through the years.

If you haven't done any flexibility training in a while, don't go overboard the first time out. You can really injure yourself if you force your joints, ligaments, and muscles to do things they aren't accustomed to doing. If you can bend over and touch your knees but go no further, then work with that. Don't force yourself to go past where you can go, and never ever bounce. It takes time to increase flexibility. Be patient with yourself and stay with your exercises.

Stretching After Aerobics

Many people think that stretching routines should be done before aerobics exercise. The exact opposite is true. Muscles must be thoroughly warmed up before you begin stretching them. If a rubber band is stretched when it is cold, it won't stretch very far before it breaks. If it is warm, however, it will stretch farther and more efficiently. The better time to stretch is at the end of a weight-training or aerobics exercise time. Stretching after active exercise minimizes spasms, promotes relaxation of the muscles as well as the mind and nervous system, and speeds recovery by minimizing the stiffness and soreness that often go along with weight-training or aerobics exercise.

Stretching and Sports

The best warm-up for any sport is to do twenty minutes of aerobics exercise and then twenty minutes of stretching exercises. Virtually any sport can be played with greater intensity if you will do these exercises *first*.

The Great Benefits of Flexibility Exercises

Stretching has a number of benefits that are not directly associated with fat loss and the building of muscle cells, but which are beneficial to your life nonetheless. Stretching gives a greater awareness of the body and helps alleviate back problems, muscle strains, and joint sprains. For women, stretching regularly often reduces the severity of painful menstruatral cramps and increases circulation. Stretching may even slow the aging process in muscles and joints.

The great benefit to fat loss is indirect. If your body remains flexible, you will feel a lot more comfort—less pained and stiff—in doing cardiovascular and strength-building exercises. In other words, you'll have a greater willingness to do the exercises that really burn up fat. If you don't remain flexible, you will want to avoid these other exercises because they will seem more difficult and painful.

Three Tips for Doing Flexibility Exercises

First, stretch your muscles in a way that protects your muscles from damage. Do not stretch your muscles to the point where you feel pain. Get into a position where the target muscle (or muscle group) feels tight but is still comfortable and hold that position for ten to fifteen seconds, then release the stretch.

Second, breathe slowly and deeply while stretching—never hold your breath.

Third, of all the stretching techniques, *static* stretching is the most popular one. It involves simply moving into a comfortable stretch and holding the position for the desired time. This is the safest technique and is the one recommended for beginners.

If you aren't sure what kinds of flexibility exercises to pursue, there are a number of books written on this topic. Check out your local bookstore. (A set of flexibility exercises can be found in the *Maximum Fat Loss Workbook*.)

STRENGTH-BUILDING EXERCISE

This type of exercise is also called resistance exercise. It is often done with weights, or by doing exercises in which your own body acts as the weight.

You need to devote at least thirty to forty-five minutes to strength-building exercises three times a week, regardless of your age. I recommend that you do this type of training every other day—which gives a day for your muscles to rebuild between workouts. If you have not worked out for several years, don't jump back in like Van. I failed to mention that after that leg workout he had a hard time walking for several days.

A study done several years ago involved a group of nursing home residents who were confined to wheelchairs. Several of these patients were able to regain enough muscle mass to leave their wheelchairs—and to enjoy light sports such as walking, golf, and softball! Few people are ever too old or sick to benefit from strength training. My mother, who is eighty-four years old, has just recently discovered the benefits of exercise.

Don't wait until you are old and atrophied to learn that this time-honored statement about your muscles is true: "If you don't use 'em, you lose 'em."

Build Muscle to Lose More Fat!

I encourage every person who embarks on a fat-loss program to think of the program as a muscle-building plan. The result of muscle-building is an increase in metabolic rate, which allows you to burn up more calories just in the course of breathing and going about your daily routine. Certainly I am not advocating that you become a bodybuilder with bulging biceps—and I especially am not advocating that for women!

Lean muscle mass, however, is absolutely necessary for efficient fat loss and the maintenance of fat loss. The achievement of lean muscle mass requires muscle growth. Even very limited amounts of strength-building exercise have been shown to increase muscle growth and overall muscle mass.

The good news is that for every pound of lean muscle mass that you build into your body, you increase your metabolic rate by about fifty calories. How does this work? It is actually a fairly simple process. It takes more calories for the body to maintain muscle tissue than fat tissue.

Also, since muscle tissue is responsible for 80 percent of the blood sugar uptake following a meal, every little bit of extra muscle gives a space for the body to store glucose and glycogen other than in fat cells!

However, if you lose muscle mass as you lose weight, you are actually going to *decrease* your metabolic rate. It's going to be increasingly more difficult for you to lose fat because your metabolism becomes slower and slower. Building and maintaining lean muscle mass is critical to achieving and then maintaining maximum fat loss.

Last year I attended an excellent medical seminar on health. During that seminar we discussed a woman named Roseanne who had lost a hundred pounds, but of that hundred, only about seventy pounds were fat. That meant she had lost about thirty pounds of muscle. In the process of losing a hundred pounds, she lowered her metabolic rate by fifteen hundred calories a day! That meant she had to eat fifteen hundred fewer calories each day just to maintain her weight. She had to consume even fewer calories to lose more weight. Eventually, a person can eat a minimal number of calories and still not lose. That's what happened to Roseanne. She had been eating only about a thousand calories a day for several weeks and hadn't lost a pound.

Had she been my client I would have immediately recommended a muscle-building plan of exercise for her. Within days, she would have started losing weight again.

It is vitally important that you build muscle even as you cut calories. There are two ways to do that, and ideally, these two ways work together: (1) exercise regularly—doing the right kinds of exercises for long enough and frequent enough periods—and (2) take supplements that can help build muscle. Some of these supplements are described in the next chapter.

STRENGTH-BUILDING IS MORE IMPORTANT THAN AEROBICS IN BURNING FAT.

Weight-training is actually *more* beneficial than cardiovascular exercise in burning fat. Mauro Di Pasquale, M.D., who has been studying the science of sports and fitness for more than three decades. He is strongly convinced that fat is burned more efficiently by a high-intensity weight training program than by aerobics.[2]

Dr. Richard Kreider, a leading sports medicine expert and professor at the University of Memphis, believes that the goal in a fat-loss program should be to burn at least three hundred calories a day through exercise. He has written, "Although any type of exercise which increases calorie expenditure is beneficial for fat loss, combining weight training—at least three hours per week—with an exercise such as sprinting appears to be very effective."[3] While I don't recommend sprinting, cardiovascular exercise will have the same effect.

Exercise all muscle groups.

Strength-building exercises should involve both fast-twitch and slow-twitch muscles. Each type of muscle fiber requires a different kind of exercise. Make sure you develop a personal program that covers both types of muscle groups. If you don't know the difference, ask an expert at your gym. I also cover this in detail in my exercise videos.

No Pain!

Do not ignore the signal of pain when doing strength-building exercises. If you feel a twinge of pain from a joint or ligament while doing a strength-training exercise, stop doing what triggered the pain. "No-pain, no gain" is not a good slogan for strength-training exercises. When I was younger, I did some strength-training exercises that were not good for my spine and joints and ultimately, I had to have back surgery that left me flat on my back for months. I didn't regain my full strength for nearly a year after that surgery. Pain in joints and ligaments is a built-in warning sign—don't ignore it. I don't recommend squats, but if you are going to do them, never use more weight than you can do in twenty-five repetitions per set. Doing heavy squats is how I hurt my back.

EXERCISE THE ENTIRE BODY

Several years ago, the National Fasteners Association flew me to northern California to speak to them about exercise and diet. Their hope was they would see a decrease in the number of sick days among their employees and also see an increase in productivity and efficiency as a result.

I was about fifteen pounds heavier than normal at the time, but I knew that. I had been travelling extensively and had not paid enough attention to my own physical needs. I have since corrected that oversight. Still, I hadn't paid much attention to just *where* this excess weight was residing in my body. As I stood before the three-way mirror in my hotel room, I had a rude awakening. I had hips! I had never stood before a three-way mirror and viewed my backside while I was unclothed. I was shocked. My hips had always been very narrow when I was working out as a young man in college. I said to my wife, Sharon, "Why didn't you tell me this was happening!"

She replied, "Well, you work out all the time and I like the way you look. I didn't see anything wrong with you."

Well, I saw something wrong! These hips of mine were completely unacceptable, even though the result was logical. As a man passes forty, testosterone begins to decline and estrogen begins to play a role. The result for men is weight distribution to areas that women often complain about. I made a new concerted effort that day to do something about the fat gain in my hips. I knew that if I didn't do something about this problem, it would only increase. It took me a while to completely eliminate the problem, but I did. That is when I started doing cardio exercises five days a week and lowered my body fat by five percent.

Part of the reason I had developed this problem also had to do with the way I had been exercising my back and hips. After rupturing the disk between my L4 and L5 vertebrae, I had become extremely cautious in the way I exercised my back and hip muscles.

A basic rule regarding exercise: Exercise the entire body. Do something about every muscle group—from the heart muscle to the abdominal muscles, from the lower back, leg, and hip muscles to the upper arm and shoulder muscles. The areas you don't exercise are the areas where your body will tend to store fat and where your muscles will start to atrophy.

INCREASE THE OVERALL ACTIVITY LEVEL OF YOUR LIFE

Aerobic, flexibility, and strength-building exercises are vital, but so is a general increase in your activity level. A good number of calories can be burned up in very simple ways:

- Take the stairs instead of the elevator or escalator at the office, in the mall, or in the department store.

- Park as far away from the entrance to the supermarket or store as possible. (In many cases, this also means less likelihood that your car will be dinged by other car doors.)

- Take a window-shopping stroll during your lunch hour. You might invite a coworker to go along. That will give you a socialization time and get you outside and moving, rather than sitting at the cafeteria table wishing you could eat a dessert with the rest of the gang.

- Choose to feed the birds in the park during your morning break or noon hour. Take birdseed with you and do something nice for creation as you walk through the park.

- If you have a choice between sitting and standing . . . stand. It burns more calories.

- Consider walking or riding a bike if you need to run errands near your home. If you have several errands in a close radius, park your car in a central location and walk to the various stores.

- Rather than walk to the refrigerator during a commercial, get on a small trampoline or a stair climber machine. Keep moving! Jogging on a small trampoline really helps to lower blood pressure and increases bone density.

Every calorie burned in movement is a calorie that isn't stored as fat!

DISPELLING THREE GREAT MYTHS ABOUT EXERCISE

Three great myths seem to surround the topic of exercise. It's time to face the truth.

"I Should Eat Something Before Exercising."

One of the big myths about exercise is that people need some type of energy food or drink before they start exercising. If your goal is to burn body fat, that is not a good idea. If you eat an energy bar or drink a high-carbohydrate sports drink before you exercise, your body will be using that fuel first. Chances are that during your workout, you won't even get to the point where you are tapping into stored body fat.

The most effective exercise for burning fat is done at least three hours *after* a person eats. One of the reasons is that the body tends to secrete even greater amount of growth hormone when you exercise several hours after a meal. Growth hormone (GH) is a potent lipolytic hormone—in other words, a fat-fighting hormone. GH is just one more reason for exercising first thing in the morning.

"I Should Eat Right After Exercise to Replenish My Body."

Your body keeps working after you stop exercising. A person is actually burning more fat just standing around after a rigorous workout than he was burning during the first fifteen minutes of exercise! Your body will continue to rely on fat stores for fuel up to an hour after you exercise.[4]

What does that mean to the person who is exercising first thing in the morning and then eating breakfast? It means simply this: Take time to cool off, shower, and get dressed and ready for the day before you eat breakfast. That time *after* your workout will allow your body to continue to burn up as much fat as possible before you introduce new fuel to your system.

"I Play a Lot of Sports So I Don't Need to Exercise."

This is sometimes stated, "I have a very physically demanding job so I don't need to exercise." Oh, but you do!

It takes a considerable amount of sports exercise to burn up calories. A 130-pound person will burn the following numbers of calories in a full hour of playing these sports:

- basketball—350
- bowling—250
- football—370
- skiing—275
- table tennis—230
- tennis—350
- volleyball—230

The most beneficial sport for burning calories is a good fast soccer game—which burns about 450 calories an hour.

Compare the previous numbers to the following:

- fast bicycling—350
- jogging—380
- running—470
- walking uphill—380
- Using the Precor EFX 544 eliptical runner—720-1000 depending on body weight

Most jobs, even heavy construction jobs, don't come anywhere close to exercising *all* parts of the body. Nor do they exercise the heart and cardiovascular system. Nor do they aid flexibility for all joints.

EIGHT IMPORTANT EXERCISE TIPS

Here are eight more tips for a personally customized exercise plan:

1. Don't Compare Yourself to Others.

Never compare yourself to another person as you pursue your exercise program at a gym or even while walking in your neighborhood.

2. Work With An Expert.

Consider the great benefits that come through working with a knowledgeable exercise physiologist or personal trainer. These professionals can help you develop a strength-training program that is custom-tailored to your body type, physiology, and personal health goals. I developed my exercise video tape series so that you can work out with me in the privacy of your own home.

3. Don't Confuse Muscle Weight With Fat Weight.

As I have said repeatedly in this book, make *fat* loss your goal, not *weight* loss. Many times people actually see a slight increase in their weight when they begin an exercise program. That's because muscle tissue is denser and heavier than body fat. You start gaining muscle weight at the same time you start burning body fat. I urge my clients to limit themselves to one trip per week to the scales. If you want to measure anything, measure body *fat loss*. That's the true measure of a "good loss."

4. Make Sure You Sleep *Well*.

Most people who engage in a regular exercise program discover that they sleep more soundly and more deeply. If that isn't your experience, take a look at the factors that may be keeping you from a good night's rest.

Recognize that your body needs an average of eight hours of sleep every twenty-four hours. Too little sleep and you are going to feel less like exercising—in fact, you are going to feel like doing less of everything! A lack of overall energy is likely to be interpreted by you as a need for more food. The fact is you don't need more food, you need more sleep and more exercise. The balance between food intake, exercise output, and good sound sleep is vital!

Your body rebuilds damaged tissues and replenishes tissue fluids and nutrients while you sleep. You need to get enough rest to help this vital rejuvenation process. If you don't sleep well at night, you will not feel rested and your body tissues will not recover properly.

Make sure you have a good mattress that is flat and firm. If your mattress sags, your spine is sagging, too! Don't scrimp when you are buying a mattress—investing in a good mattress is investing in your health.

Sleep on your side. I recommend the use of three pillows—one between your legs, one underneath your arm, and one for your head. Avoid overstuffed pillows. Your head and neck should remain at an angle close to their normal position so you don't get a kinked neck. I personally use a buckwheat-filled pillow for maximum support. (Those with dust allergies should avoid down or feather pillows.)

A bad night's sleep can leave you with sore muscles, stiffness, and discomfort. A good night's sleep can leave you feeling energized, vital, and healthy. The true fountain of youth is likely to be a good night's sleep and a healthy day's eating, drinking, and exercising.

5. Have the right gear.

I'm not talking about buying gimmick products (which includes most of those you see on television infomercials). You need to have the best gear for doing the exercises you are doing—aerobics, flexibility exercises, and strength-building exercises.

Always wear appropriate shoes for exercising—walking shoes for walking, dancing shoes for dancing, jogging or running shoes for jogging or running. Good padding and support can help you avoid injuries and make the entire exercise experience more enjoyable.

Anticipate rain and cold weather. Have a rain parka. Dress in layers that you can put on and peel off. Refuse to allow weather to become an excuse for not exercising. If you usually engage in an outdoor activity, plan an alternate indoor activity for those days when the weather is bad.

If you are exercising before dawn, or after dark, be sure you can be seen by others. Wear reflective tape or clothing. White or light colors are best.

If you are a swimmer, wear goggles to protect your eyes from the chlorine. You might also want to get a pair of ear plugs.

If you are a cyclist, be sure to wear a helmet and protection for knees and elbows. The same for those of you who are roller-bladers.

Make sure your exercise clothing gives you plenty of room for flexing muscles and doing a wide range of motion.

Have the equipment you need to make your work-outs *safe* and *comfortable*. Most gear is sold to make you look stylish. That's nice, even fun, but not necessary.

6. Exercise With Others.

Make your morning exercise time a family time. Get your spouse and teenagers out there walking or jogging with you. If you're out early on the weekends, make your morning a time for a family bike ride or a family swim. Not only can this be a time for family fun and communication, but you will be building an exercise habit into your children.

I strongly encourage you to have at least one family tradition that involves physical exertion. Several times a year my wife and my oldest child, Austin, and I go to the Great Smokey Mountain National Park near Gatlinburg, Tennessee, to hike Mount LeConte. It's an eleven-mile hike that challenges all of us—a great cardiovascular workout. I especially recommend the Alum Cave Bluff trail. I've been hiking Mount LeConte for twenty-seven years now, and I'm planning on hiking it for another fifty years . . . with my wife and all three of my children as they become old enough for the trek, and someday with my grandchildren and perhaps even great-grandchildren!

If you don't have a family or if family members won't join you, find a friend who will! Agree to motivate each other. Make an exercise commitment that you will encourage each other if one of you feels like sleeping in or taking a week off.

If you don't have a friend . . . join a gym! Don't worry about what you look like the first day you go. So what if you don't look all that great in shorts! That's today. You'll look increasingly better as the days and weeks pass! You can always wear sweatpants and a sweatshirt. I love wearing these. They really help me to warm up and stay warm through the workout.

7. Double Task.

This is a suggestion for all of you who feel that exercise is a time waster. Choose to use your exercise time for mental problem-solving, even if its just what to buy your child as a present for his next birthday or where to go on your next vacation.

If you feel deprived of the news, watch the news while you ride an exercise bike or walk on a treadmill.

I know a man who taught himself French over a two-year period of walking. He listened to language tapes every morning, just twenty minutes a day. Yet another client of mine listens to the latest novel on tape as she walks every morning. She's always up on the latest best-sellers.

I also recommend health and fitness audio tapes—they help boost your motivate to continue your exercise program.[5]

8. Have Fun!

Choose to have fun while you exercise. If walking or jogging around a track or your neighborhood isn't much fun for you, do something to make it fun. Try listening to music you like or to tapes that are inspiring, even informative. I know one woman who loves to walk to a tape of Souza marches. It brings back good memories of high-school marching-band days and helps her keep up a good pace to her walking so she doesn't slow to a stroll.

Or, find an early-morning swimmercize class if you'd like a group experience for low-impact aerobics. Or, go to a gym with an indoor pool so you can swim laps before heading toward the office. If you like to dance, put on your shoes and do your own aerobics dancing.

If you get bored doing one kind of exercise after a while, switch to another. Losing interest in exercise is often a sign of overtraining. If you've been riding a bike, try walking. If you've been walking, try swimming.

Make your exercise time interesting—make it something you look forward to doing every day!

Make sure you are careful. If you decide to engage in a high-risk activity for exercise you are probably going to have to deal with injuries. These injuries could force you to take an extended lay off. That is why I am so careful in the gym and rarely engage in activities other than the Precor and lifting weights.

BUILDING EXERCISE INTO YOUR DAILY ROUTINE

Are you procrastinating in starting an exercise program or in changing the way you eat? Few of us do everything we would like to do, but procrastination is a chronic wait-until-tomorrow state of being. The fact is, for the procrastinator, tomorrow never comes.

Anybody can miss a workout or two, but if a week goes by and you fail to break a sweat . . . you're a procrastinator.

Anybody can have a good excuse for missing a workout, but if your reasons for not exercising are becoming more and more complicated or creative . . . you're a procrastinator. Finding the perfect shorts to match your walking shoes is not a good reasons for failing to exercise. Shift your imagination toward how to make exercise more fun!

If you are spending more and more time thinking about exercising and less and less time actually exercising . . . you are a procrastinator. Procrastinators often feel discomfort or uneasiness about something they are avoiding. Remove that discomfort from your mind and put on your walking shoes.

The good news about procrastination is that it can be overcome without taking any supplements or consulting any experts. The common phrase, "Just do it" is what's needed. Figure out how to motivate yourself to become the healthiest person you can possibly be, not only today but for all your life. Nobody will ever be able to motivate you into action better than you can motivate yourself to action.

Those who actually start exercising are likely to feel like continuing to exercise.

Finding Time in Your Schedule

Every person on the planet has these things in common: We each must breathe, drink water, eat, and sleep periodically, and we each have 1,440 minutes in a day. I remind people of this every time they try to tell me they are too busy to eat the right things, drink pure water, or exercise.

You must eat anyway; you may as well eat the right things. You must drink water; why not make sure it's pure and that you are drinking enough?

You must sleep; it's to your benefit to get *enough* sleep. Sleep deprivation for most people translates into counter-productiveness. Those who are sleep-deprived very often have to do things twice to get them right. Tasks take longer, a lack of ability to concentrate and focus results in more mistakes, and an irritable mood can produce more and more reasons for needing to apologize and made amends with those around you.

When I was in graduate school at Florida State University, I learned that it was far better for me to get a good night's sleep before a big exam than to stay up most of the night studying. When you are exhausted, you make ridiculous mistakes, not only on exams, but in *life*.

You must move or your muscles will atrophy; why not move your muscles in ways that generate health and help with fat loss!

All of which is to say; "Yes, you do have time for exercise." If you have to, give up something else in order to have that time. Let's face it. If you don't take time for your health and fitness they will decline.

FIVE TIPS FOR FINDING TIME TO EXERCISE

Where can you find the time for exercise every day. Here are my Top Five Tips for carving out an exercise period each day. They are also tips that just might increase the quality of your overall life along the way.

1. Watch Less Television.

TV is the biggest time vampire in our culture. The average American spends thirty hours a week watching TV, and the vast majority of Americans would argue vigorously that they just can't find four hours a week to exercise! For the most part, people can't tell you what they watched on television five nights ago. Even more sadly, they can't tell you why what they saw is important to their lives. Do you really need to know the weather report in a state five hundred miles away or whether a train accident occurred in Lower Slobovia?

2. Eliminate Mindless Phone Chatter.

In any given day, most people blow at least an hour on chitchat. This is even true in the business world. Personal phone conversations are almost as bad as television when it comes to consuming time and giving little to show for it. If you insist on spending time on the phone, do so only as you walk on a treadmill or ride a stationary bike. At least you'll be accomplishing something productive. I have several friends who spend thousands of minutes on cell phones each month. (They use the hands-free head sets.) None of these friends has any time for exercise. I wonder why.

3. Make a List of Daily Things To Do That Includes Exercise.

Every night write down those things that you want to accomplish the next day. Review your list to make sure these are things that are really important to your accomplishing your big goals in life. I put "work out," "go to church," "take supplements," "spend time with family," and "eat six meals" on my list. Keep your list with you all the next day and check off things as you complete them.

Remember to cluster your errands on a given day in a certain area of town. So many people drive all over town forgetting to do some small item while they are there making it necessary for them to drive back. This not only wastes fuel and time it is very inefficient for your schedule.

Two things happen when you do this. One, you'll find that you get more done. Many people waste time reacting, adjusting, and trying to figure out what to do, when to do it, or how to do it. If you plan ahead, you know what you're going to do and when you're going to do it. Very often just planning in advance gives you time to figure out how to do it by the time the actual "doing time" comes around.

Second, you'll find that marking off the things you've done gives you a sense of accomplishment. This sense of accomplishment is a form of self-reward. There's satisfaction to be gained by crossing off "work out" on any given day.

It only takes a few minutes to map out a day and you'll likely find that the day runs more smoothly if you have a list to guide you. In fact, you'll very likely find more than enough time for a workout.

4. Eat out less often.

If you eat out at restaurants more than a once a week, cut back. The time you'll save waiting to be served what is often a high-calorie meal can be put to better use.

A number of people have told me through the years that it takes too much time for them to prepare nutritious meals. That may have been true twenty or thirty years ago, but not today. It takes very little time to make a protein shake in the morning—usually less time than it takes to order, pay your money, and get your food at a fast-food restaurant's drive-through. That one protein shake can be two of your six meals.

At times my family and I have spent upwards of an hour waiting to be seated, putting in our order from a menu, and then being served in a restaurant. In just one hour, a bag of greens can be chopped for several days worth of salads, a platter of chicken can be grilled or baked for later use, and baggies of fresh vegetables can be prepared for snacks. In other words, *several* days worth of meals can be prepared in just one hour.

5. Get To Bed a Half Hour Earlier.

Many people have discovered that for every half hour of sleep they get before midnight, they need an hour's less sleep for the entire night. The sleep you get before midnight seems to do more for you— it's generally the most peaceful and rejuvenating sleep you get. By getting to bed a half hour earlier, you should be able to get up a half hour to an hour earlier in the morning. There's your exercise time! Let me ask you a question. Do you really have to hear the late news? Or is this just a habit that you could easily break?

You'll Get the Time Back.

I firmly believe that if you exercise four to five hours a week, you are going to find that you have more energy for everything else you desire to do—so much more energy, in fact, that other chores and tasks are going to get done a lot more quickly than before.

Exercise seems to yield a double dividend—for every hour I exercise, I seem to get back an extra two hours a week through increased efficiency and productivity in my performance of other tasks.

Build exercise into your schedule right along with your daily devotional time. It's that important.

TAKE AN *ACTION* STEP

At the beginning of this book, we talked about the importance of taking an action step. When it comes to exercise, I mean that literally. Start moving!

Get up right now and go for a walk! Only take time to put on suitable walking shoes. You may move only at stroll pace, but *move*.

When you get back from your walk, look up gyms in your phone book and make a call to set up an appointment to visit one. Start checking out a good place for strength-building exercise. Ask about group aerobics classes.

Then get out your daily planner and start marking in exercise times.

There's no time like the present!

KEY #12:

Take supplements daily to help you fight fat and give your body all the nutrients it needs.

17

THE SUPPLEMENTS YOU NEED TO FIGHT THE FAT WAR

Does the average person need supplemental nutrients? Without a doubt. Food just doesn't provide all the nutrients a person needs, especially the nutrients a person needs to lose fat.

The human body needs forty-five essential nutrients for good health. These are nutrients that must be taken into the body from an outside source. Of these forty-five nutrients, twenty are minerals, fifteen are vitamins, eight are essential amino acids (building blocks for proteins), and two are essential fatty acids. We need sufficient quantities of these nutrients every day for optimal health and maximum fat loss.

A large-scale government survey has shown that more than 60 percent of the North American population is deficient in one or more of ten nutrients evaluated. If 60 percent are deficient in that small sampling of nutrients, I can only guess what percentage would be deficient if the other essential nutrients were also studied!

"But I eat a balanced diet."

I have heard that statement more times than I can count. When I ask a person to document what precisely they eat—recording every morsel of food on a food diary, including the amount of each item eaten—they are usually amazed at how unbalanced their diet really is.

A balanced diet over the course of six meals a day is only a beginning to a truly adequate intake of nutrients. The hard cold fact is this: Today's genetically-engineered, chemical-laden, pesticide-riddled, chemically-fertilized, and totally processed food doesn't meet the basic vitamin and mineral needs of the average person.

Part of the reason for this is that our soil no longer has the mineral content it once had. Early harvesting of produce—which is passed on to us unripened or ripened as the result of chemical vapors—takes away some of the nutritional value. Processing gets rid of many nutrients. And then, most of us overcook our food and boil away most of the remaining nutritional value! In my *Eat, Drink and Be Healthy* program I go into detail on proper food selection, preparation, and how to do the best you can with today's food selections. Remember: *Do not buy genetically engineered food!*

You also need to recognize that changes in your exercise and eating patterns creates a different level of need for certain nutrients.

For example, strenuous exercise actually causes calcium retention in the body and has a positive effect. However, exercise and stress also cause the body to lose chromium, copper, iron, selenium, zinc, and magnesium.[1]

As another example, many vegetables—especially the leafy green vegetables recommended for a fat-loss plan—have high levels of some minerals. A high phytate content of these vegetables, which refers to a form of phosphorus found in fiber, may limit the absorption of the minerals. Phytates, which are also found in cereals and grains, especially inhibit the absorption of zinc.

Recommended Dietary Allowances

"But my vitamin and mineral tablet claims to give me most of the recommended dietary allowance (RDA)," you may say.

All vitamin and mineral tablets and capsules are labeled according to the percentage of the Recommended Dietary Allowances (RDA) they offer. But what do these numbers mean?

The RDA is published by the Food and Nutrition Board of the National Research Council. Many of the participants in the council believe that RDAs no longer make up for deficiencies in peoples' diets, however. In most cases, the RDA is well below what a body actually needs.

RDAs also do not take into consideration the age of a person taking the vitamin or mineral. In reviewing the vitamin requirements of older people, a Tufts University research team concluded that the 1989 RDAs may be too low for B2, B6, B12, and vitamin D, and too high for vitamin A.[2]

RDAs also do not take into consideration the weight of the person taking the pill. Those who are obese usually need more than the recommended amounts.

Personally, I believe RDA should stand for "ridiculous daily amounts"— the amounts are so low that every nutritionist I know considers them to be ludicrous.

A one-a-day chemical vitamin or metallic mineral pill is not sufficient. You cannot buy a pill big enough to contain all you need. Plus the majority of these products are less than you need because of their low quality shellac coating and non-absorbing processing. The key to supplementation is *adequate amounts.*

A simple hair analysis is often the easiest way of determining whether you have any mineral deficiencies. You may contact my office for more information on this.[3]

Mineral deficiencies, even more than vitamin deficiencies, can be directly related to weight gain. Certain minerals that I discussed earlier are key for proper glucose metabolism.

Three General Words of Caution

As important as it is to take supplements, let me give you three general words of caution at the outset of our discussion.

1. With the exception of vitamin C and other water-soluable

vitamins, do *not* take megadoses of any supplement for a prolonged period of time without consulting a trained professional. You want an *adequate* amount of nutrients, but not prolonged megadoses!

2. Do *not* expect fat-burning supplements alone to do all of the work. Too many people buy into products and supplements that claim to "burn off the fat" while you sit and do nothing. The result of this approach is zero. In fact, you are likely to be doing your body harm. Fat-burning supplements only work properly if your exercise and nutrition program is in line.

3. Avoid any tendency to skip a workout or blow your eating plan and then just take supplements. Again, that's not the way these supplements work. They are a boost for a good exercise and nutrition program, but never a replacement for a good, clean diet, intense workouts, and sufficient water to keep the body flushed of any toxins that may be generated as a by-product of fat-burning processes.

NUTRIENTS THAT HELP WITH FAT LOSS

Nutritional supplements that help with fat loss tend to fall into three general categories:

I. Nutrients That Reduce Water Retention

These nutrients and diuretic herbs flush water out of the body, creating a loss of water weight. This is not true fat loss and should never be considered as such. Many fad diets offer the opportunity to lose up to ten pounds in just a few days. They do this by removing water from the tissues and bloodstream. Then, when a person quits taking the diuretics, the weight reappears. That's not healthful for the body, nor is it genuine fat loss.

The body does, however, need to flush itself with water. Nutrients that reduce water retention can be important in assisting the body in the transportation of fat globules from the bloodstream so they do not stick or plaque onto arterial walls. Sufficient water intake is critically important to the person who begins a fat-loss plan. If you do not take in sufficient water, the body will store the water it has and it will also keep any fat that is released into the bloodstream. Arteries are *not* a good place for fat to be deposited! For further details on water systems please call my office.

2. Nutrients That Reduce Cholesterol and Fat

This class of nutrients is called lipotropic vitamins. They work to break down cholesterol and fat into molecules that can be flushed away from the body.

3. Nutrients That Are Natural Appetite-Suppressants

These nutrients tend to make a person feel full and satisfied so that carbohydrate craving is averted. Most of these products are fiber in nature. They bond with fat in the digestive tract and help remove fat from the colon (reducing the risk of colon cancer in the process). They help the body maintain regular elimination of toxins, including fat.

Ask about any supplement that you put into your body: "What is this supposed to do in my body?" Know what you are taking, and why.

TED'S TOP TEN FAT-LOSS SUPPLEMENTS

Here are my top ten picks of fat-loss nutrients that can be taken in supplemental form. Some of them may be grouped together in various products that may be available in a quality nutrition store.[4] If you are unable to find them please call my office. For each supplement, I have noted what the supplement does along with the recommended dosage.

1. Chromium Picolinate

Chromium has been shown to reduce sugar cravings by stabilizing the metabolism of simple carbohydrates. It is an extremely valuable supplement for those with diabetes or hypoglycemia because it helps to regulate blood sugar levels. Normal dosage is two hundred to six hundred micrograms daily.

Both soy protein and chromium (chromium picolinate and chromium polynicotinate) appear to have a positive influence on insulin sensitivity.[5]

Chromium supplementation has been linked to improvements in insulin use and a lowering of serum lipids, including the high-density lipoprotein cholesterol.[6] The need for chromium increases with exercise and some studies have shown that a chromium deficiency may be relatively common among those who exercise regularly.[7]

Chromium (as well as copper) should be taken on an empty stomach between breakfast and lunch. A dose of one hundred to two hundred micrograms of chromium and two to four milligrams of copper is usually sufficient. Copper, by the way, helps to maintain the elasticity of blood vessels.

Chromium (as well as vanadium) deficiencies result in an intense craving for carbohydrates. Chromium, and vanadyl sulfate supplements are usually a part of a trace-mineral supplement program and can be vital in helping a person control these urges for carbohydrate consumption.

2. Lecithin

This can be purchased in granule or capsule form. Lecithin is a fat emulsifier—in other words, it breaks down fat so it can be readily removed from the body. If you are using granules, take one tablespoon three times a day before meals. In capsule form, the dosage is 1,200 milligrams three times a day before meals.

The best source of lecithin is soybean oil. Lecithin is found in every cell of your body and about 17 to 20 percent of the brain is made from lecithin. Lecithin keeps fat moving. It is a natural diuretic and an effective cholesterol-reducer. In addition, it's a great source of two of the hardest-to-find B vitamins: choline and inositol. Not only that, it's loaded with vitamin E.

You can buy lecithin in granule or powder form to be mixed with other foods or into protein drinks. It comes in capsules or chewable tablets as well. My wife and I use the granular lecithin daily—we simply add it to our protein shakes.

3. L-Arginine

L-Arginine, along with L-Ornithine and L-Lysine (described below), plus a fifty miligram tablet of vitamin B6 and a 100 milligram tablet of vitamin C makes an excellent "bedtime cocktail" of nutrients that are especially beneficial in helping your body burn fat all night long!

Take five hundred milligrams of L-Arginine, or as directed on the label, before bedtime on an empty stomach with water or juice. Do not use milk with this amino acid. It needs to be taken with L-Lysine. You'll find that this amino acid is better absorbed if you take it with fifty miligrams of vitamin B6 and one hundred milligrams of vitamin C.

L-Arginine should not be used by those who have diabetes, ocular or brain herpes infections, pituitary dysfunction, or cancer.

4. L-Ornithine

Take five hundred milligrams or as directed on the label. Take before bedtime, with water or juice, on an empty stomach. Do not take with milk. Take it with L-Lysine, fifty milligrams of vitamin B6 and one hundred milligrams of vitamin C.

L-Ornithine should not be used by those who have diabetes, ocular or brain herpes infections, pituitary dysfunction, or cancer.

5. L-Lysine

Again, take five hundred milligrams or as directed on the label. Take before bedtime on an empty stomach with water or juice, and with fifty milligrams of vitamin B6 and one hundred milligrams of vitamin C. Do not take with milk or if you are diabetic.

6. L-Carnitine

This amino acid, which is found in many foods and especially in meat, helps ensure optimal metabolism of fat. It has the ability to break up fat deposits and it aids in weight loss. It is an especially important supplement to consider if your fat loss is exceeding one and a half pounds a week.

If you take it in supplement form, be sure to take it with meals. Recommended dosage is five hundred milligrams daily.

Make certain that you take L-Carnitine. The use of D-Carnitine or D-L-Carnitine has been associated with some severe side effects. Check the label!

I suggest you use caution in taking L-Carnitine. It causes me to have headaches after several days. It probably is a supplement better taken every other day, or in cycles.

7. L-Glutamine

L-Glutamine is not to be confused with the toxic glutamic acid. L-Glutamine reduces carbohydrate cravings. Use as directed on the label.

L-Glutamine nourishes the cells of the immune system in important ways. It is an essential nitrogen transporter that allows ammonia to be removed from the body, specifically from the brain and lungs. Glutamine is one of the main building blocks in most powerful antioxidant produced in the body: gluthathione (made from glutamine, cysteine, and glycine).[8]

Of all the amino acids, glutamine appears to be by far the most important one in helping muscle cells to stay hydrated and continue to grow (as opposed to becoming dehydrated, shriveled, and wasting away).

Sufficient glutamine is a basic necessity for good protein synthesis, too. In all, it's a powerful supplement.

The best time to take glutamine is right after exercise. Alanine seems to help preserve muscle glutamine concentrations, and glycine, in combination with glutamine, induces cell-volumizing effects that are significantly greater than those generated by glutamine alone.

I add this nutrient daily to my protein shake.

8. Zinc

Zinc enhances the effectiveness of insulin and boosts the immune system. Use zinc gluconate for best absorption. My recommended dosage is sixty milligrams a day, but do not exceed a total of one hundred milligrams daily from all supplements. Check the label on your general mineral supplement. If eighty milligrams of zinc are included, do not add additional zinc.

The general symptoms related to zinc and magnesium deficiency are general fatigue, muscle weakness, lowered sperm count, slow wound healing, suppressed immunity, loss of appetite, lowered sex drive in men, and in severe cases, nausea and mental confusion. If you experience these symptoms, you might try zinc and magnesium supplements.

Zinc should be taken on an empty stomach at night before bedtime. Both of these minerals may also enhance the release of growth hormones.

I recommend approximately 60 milligrams of zinc. Zinc is water-soluble and therefore, if too much is taken, it is easily excreted in the urine. Most Americans take far too little zinc into their bodies on a daily basis. Foods are deficient in zinc in today's world because much of the zinc in our soil has been leached away through years of farming. Processing removes the richest sources of zinc—the germ and bran of grains. Cooking dissolves the mineral. And foods that contain chemicals such as EDTA, a chelating agent, remove the mineral.

Adequate zinc is necessary for many functions associated with the absorption of nutrients and the digestive processes of the body. Zinc is an important antioxidant as well, especially for diabetics. And it promotes healing, tissue repair, and muscle growth.[9]

Zinc must be taken in proportionate levels to copper, iron, and chromium. The product I take balances zinc with copper, iron, and chromium. Negative side effects related to zinc only tend to occur in large doses, generally more than 150 milligrams a day.[10]

By the way, if a man takes sixty milligrams of zinc daily, plus 1,600 IU of natural vitamin E, he will probably find that his libido (sex drive) is greatly enhanced. In addition, zinc raises sperm count.[11]

9. Magnesium

If you find on your new fat-loss program that you seem low on energy, check your magnesium consumption. Most people feel increased energy after only four or five days of magnesium supplementation, but for some people, up to two weeks is necessary before they feel renewed energy. One study in England showed that seven out of fifteen patients who suffered from chronic fatigue syndrome reported increased energy after receiving magnesium injections.

Magnesium is related to more than three hundred different chemical reactions in the body. The mitochondria, which are responsible for energy production, depend heavily on it. Magnesium also promotes muscle strength, endurance, and relaxation. It is vitally important for protein synthesis.[12]

Like zinc, magnesium may enhance release of growth hormone, which is important for building muscle.

Magnesium deficiency has been linked to heart disease. In fact, if you or a loved one ever experience a heart attack, I recommend that you ask for a magnesium injection. These injections have been shown to be highly beneficial to those experiencing heart attacks, although many physicians don't know about them.

Make sure your eating plan includes foods rich in magnesium, such as whole grains, beans, sesame seeds, and a limited quantity of nuts (such as blanched almonds and cashews). Halibut and sole are fish high in magnesium. Avocados are also a great source of this mineral.

Magnesium supplements are also available. You should go easy on supplements at first because, in excessive amounts, they can cause diarrhea. Stay away from cheaper, inorganic forms such as magnesium chloride or carbonate. Instead, take the supplements that have the words malate, fumarate, citrate, taurate, or glycinate associated with magnesium—these forms are better absorbed, tolerated, and utilized in the body.

I recommend four hundred to five hundred milligrams of magnesium. It should be taken on an empty stomach at night before bedtime.

Magnesium is a mineral that works in balance with calcium. Too much calcium can block magnesium absorption. Vitamin B6 works with magnesium in many of the energy-producing reactions.

An aluminum build-up in the body lessens the effectiveness of magnesium. Some areas of the United States with "hard water" treat their water with sodium aluminate to prevent a build-up of calcium and magnesium deposits in the water pipes. This can also lead to an aluminum build-up in the body. I believe aluminum buildup is a major factor in Alzheimer's disease.

Antiperspirants are also a source of aluminum build-up. A few years ago, the players of the Seattle Supersonics basketball team were found to have an elevation of aluminum and a deficiency of magnesium. The researchers who made this discovery also noted that most of these players were using antiperspirants that contained aluminum chlorohydrate. The solution? Switch from using an anti-perspirant to using a simple deodorant. These are usually found only in a health food store.

10. Hydroxycitric Acid (HCA)

This substance is extracted from the rind of the fruit of the *Garcinia cambogia* tree. Not only does HCA suppress hunger but it helps to prevent the body from turning carbohydrate calories into fat. It does this by inhibiting the action of an enzyme called ATP-citrate lyase. HCA is an ingredient in a number of diet products but you can also buy it in supplement form. Follow the directions on the label.

NOT IN THE TOP TEN, BUT GOOD!

Among the supplements that may show good benefit in weight loss are the following:

Conjugated Linoleic Acid

Conjugated linoleic acid (CLA) has been shown to help burn body fat. It is a naturally occurring fatty acid that helps to support healthy glucose and insulin metabolism. In other words, it helps to stabilize blood sugar and in doing so helps the body burn fat. I take 4000 milligrams daily and highly recommend it.

Xylitol

This is a low-glycemic carbohydrate that has been shown in some studies to help the body burn fat for fuel over and above even blood sugar.[13]

Synephrine

This substance has been called the calmer chemical cousin to ephedrine. The supplement seems to offer many of the metabolic-enhancing effects of ephedrine without the side effects (such as the jitters). It seems to work best when combined with tyrosine.

L-Tyrosine

This amino acid is the basic nutrient used by the body to make 90 percent of the brain's neurotransmitters, the "messengers" that carry signals between brain cells. Neurotransmitters carry the messages that tell your muscles to flex and contract. The stronger the signal, the stronger your muscle's perform. It also helps promote alertness without any unwanted central-nervous-system side effects—in other words, without that wired or "jazzed up" feeling.

Do not take L-Tyrosine, however, if you use MAO inhibitors, have cardiac arrhythmias, psychosis, preexisting malignant melanoma-type cancer, or have a violent temper.

HMB (B–hydroxy B–methyl butyrate monohydrate)

This is one of the most studied products available. It is a patented amino acid metabolite discovered by research scientists at Iowa State University. HMB boosts the stamina of athletes and helps build muscle and burn fat by minimizing protein breakdown during intense exercise. If you are diligent in cutting your calories and exercising hard, your fat-loss program may be benefited by supplementing your diet with up to three grams of HMB a day.

Creatine Monohydrate

Creatine is yet another substance that has been shown to increase the body's metabolic rate and help the body burn more calories.[14] It is also a cell volumizer and helps to increase lean muscle mass. It should however be cycled and not taken for prolonged periods of time. Remember, as a cell volumizer, it will cause water-weight gain.

Calcium

Calcium helps in activating lipase, an enzyme that breaks down fats for use by the body. Recommended dosage is 1,500 milligrams daily. Calcium needs to be taken in balance with magnesium.[15]

Boron

The U.S. Department of Agriculture concluded in a 1994 study that the trace mineral boron may speed up the burning of calories. Raisins and onions are good food sources of boron. (Raisins can be high in calories but just a few as part of a meal are acceptable.) Boron is available in supplement form. It also seems to increase testosterone production.

HERBS THAT HELP WITH FAT LOSS

In addition to the nutrients described above, there are eight general categories of herbs, or herb products, that you may find useful in your fat-loss program. I've tried to group some of them together according to their general function.

Herbal Diuretic Teas

Alfalfa, corn silk, dandelion, gravel root, horsetail, hydrangea, hyssop, juniper berries, oat straw, parsley, seawrack, thyme, uva ursi, white ash, and yarrow can be used in tea form as natural diuretics.

Aloe Vera

This juice improves digestion and cleanses the digestive tract. Aloe vera-based products can often help with constipation. I use a product called Atri Aloe. It helps to keep the colon clean, reduces in the risk of colon cancer and eliminates constipation in most people. It is not addictive.

Herbs That Aid Digestion

Butcher's broom, cardamon, cayenne, cinnamon, *Garcinia cambogia*, ginger, green tea, and mustard seed are thermogenic herbs. They improve digestion and aid in the metabolism of fat. Do not use cinnamon, however, in large quantities if you are pregnant or think you might become pregnant.

Herbs That Improve Thyroid Function

Bladderwrack, borage seed, hawthorn berry, and sarsaparilla stimulate the adrenal glands and improve thyroid function. Kelp tablets have also been known to improve thyroid production because of their iodine content.

Fennel

Fennel removes mucus and fat from the intestinal tract and is a natural appetite suppressant.

Fenugreek

This herb helps dissolve fat in the liver.

Siberian Ginseng

This herb aids in moving fluids and nutrients throughout the body and reduces the stress often associated with acquiring new eating habits. A word of caution, however. Do not use this herb if you have hypoglycemia, high blood pressure, or a heart disorder.

Herbs That Suppress Appetite

Ephedra, guarana, and kola nut are appetite suppressants. Be very caution in using ephedra, however. Do not use ephedra if you suffer from anxiety, glaucoma, heart disease, high blood pressure, or insomnia, or if you are taking an MAO inhibiter for depression. Ephedra is dangerous—be very careful. If you feel it is absolutely necessary, use it only every other day. Guarana and Kola nut also contain caffeine.

Three That Have a Reputation for Fat-Burning

Let me call your attention to three herbs that have received a lot of press as fat-loss aids.

Ephedrine. Ephedrine, also known as *ma huang,* suppresses the appetite. It has thermogenic effects, especially when combined with caffeine and aspirin. Most of ephedrine's side effects dissipate within a short time and it has an advantage over PPA in its ability to spare lean tissue (including muscle). Some reports, however, have linked ephedrine to both strokes and high blood pressure in susceptible people or those who overdose. *Ephedrine is not safe for everyone.* Those with preexisting conditions including prostate enlargement, cardiovascular disease, thyroid diseases, and diabetes should not use it. Those who are prone to depression should only use ephedrine with great caution.

The effects of ephedrine are directly correlated to the number of calories a person is eating. On a low-calorie diet, forty milligrams of ephedrine was shown to be more effective than twenty milligrams. However, the reverse was true when subjects consumed a higher-calorie diet. In other words, you can't eat anything you want and pop ephedrine and expect to lose weight.[16]

Ephedrine is banned in several states but its herbal parent, ephedra—or *ma huang,* as it's known in the Orient—is still widely available. Ephedra teas have been used for centuries in the Orient in a way similar to our use of coffee or black tea for a morning or late-afternoon pick-me-up.

Ephedra is an herb that should not be overused and should never be used if you experience heart palpitations, elevations in blood pressure, or headaches. Again, be careful. This stuff can be *dangerous!* If you are going to use this regardless of how much I have warned you, use a stacked product in capsule form that contains a powder. This way you do not have to take an entire capsule. Use only one quarter of the contents of the powder in a capsule to start with, and do not use it every day. Take this before a workout, on an empty stomach with a large glass of purified water. I occasionally take this product before a hard workout, but encourage you to remember the side effect warnings. Also remember that my blood pressure is normally 118 over 68. Be careful.

Yohimbe Bark Extract. This is an herbal extract of the bark of an African tree. This substance seems to help sexual function in men, but in women, the herb seems to decrease fat synthesis and increase the release of fatty acids from fat stores.[17]

St. John's Wort. This has been shown to extend the life of neu-rotransmitters. It may decrease food cravings and help a person avoid food binges.

Four Additional Plant Products to Consider

These products are not classified as herbs, per se, but rather, as foods that can assist in fat loss. They generally work to supply fiber and detoxify the body, in addition to providing valuable nutrients:

Chlorella. Chlorella—a small, one-celled algae—is a power-house of vitamins, minerals, and protein. It contains more chloro-phyll than any other edible plant and has 60 percent good-quality protein. It is an excellent product to take to help detoxify your body. It should be taken with at least eight ounces of water. Use it accord-ing to instructions on the product you purchase.

Wheat Grass. Wheat grass is high in fiber and protein. It con-tains chlorophyll and other nutrients that are often associated with deep green and leafy vegetables. When taken before meals with a large glass of water, wheat grass expands at least fifteen times its orig-inal volume to help a person feel full. Wheat grass tablets do not con-tain sugar. The product usually comes in tables or wafers. Use according to manufacturer's instructions. I use this regularly.

Barley. Young barley can be juiced to yield a product that is a rich source of vitamins, minerals, and enzymes. It is especially rich in vitamins B1 and B12 and is high in vitamin C, carotene, and calcium. It is also found in tablets or granules. Use according to manufac-turer's instructions.

Kelp. Kelp acts on obesity by helping to normalize thyroid gland function. It also has a normalizing effect on the nervous system, arteries, colon, liver, gall bladder, and metabolism related to fat cells.

Do not try to treat yourself for an underactive or overactive thy-roid condition with kelp. Talk to your physician first. He or she may prescribe thyroid medication.

Sodium Pyruvate. If your physician is savvy about nutrition, he may talk to you about taking sodium pyruvate (and at the same time, increasing your potassium).

When thyroid hormone is low in the bloodstream, two mechanisms seem to be at work. One is associated with low levels of adenosine triphosphate (ATP), the energy source for transferring glucose into liver cells. A way to increase ATP levels is by taking dietary pyruvate—the gateway compound for activating the Krebs (or citric acid) Cycle that produces ATP. Many compounds are involved in the Krebs cycle, but the starting point is pyruvate. Dietary pyruvate is available in the form of a mineral salt—sodium pyruvate.

A key research study was done in this area by Dr. Ronald Stanko at the University of Pittsburgh. Dietary sodium pyruvate increased aerobic performance and caused a greater fat loss at a dosage of twenty-eight grams of pyruvate a day. Since that amount of pyruvate adds more than seven grams of sodium to the body, additional potassium must also be taken to offset the sodium increase.

Lately, Dr. Stanko has been recommending five grams a day of pyruvate. Even with this lower dosage, be sure to take additional potassium.[18] Because of the high sodium levels I do not use this product.

GENERAL SUPPLEMENTS THAT ARE VERY HELPFUL

I would be remiss if I didn't mention several other very helpful nutrients that can be taken in supplement form. A mounting pile of scientific research is showing that vitamins, especially vitamin E and vitamin C, beta carotene, and minerals such as zinc and selenium, may offer significant protection against cancer, atherosclerosis, birth defects, cataracts, and other conditions.

Vitamins also have impact on fat loss in these ways:

Vitamin C with Bioflavonoids

Vitamin C actually helps to speed up a slow metabolism, prompting the body to burn more calories. It also assists in normal glandular function. The general recommended dosage for those on a fat-loss program is three thousand to six thousand milligrams daily. Space out your vitamin C. I recommend taking a thousand milligrams with each of your six meals every day.

Vitamin B Complex

The B vitamins help greatly to promote good digestion. The recommended dosage is fifty milligrams three times a day. Riboflavin (B2) helps the body to be more efficient in burning calories. You may want to take an extra fifty milligrams three times a day beyond what is in the fifty milligrams B complex. Niacin (B3) reduces sugar cravings and it can also be taken as fifty milligrams three times a day—but do not exceed this amount and do not take niacin if you have a liver disorder, gout, or high blood pressure. Vitamin B6 boosts the metabolism. An additional five hundred milligrams three times a day is helpful. The same for vitamin B12—fifty milligrams three times a day—to help in proper digestion and absorption.

Choline and inositol are part of the B-vitamin family. Both of these help the body burn fat and can often be purchased as separate supplements. Use as directed on the label of the product you purchase.

SUPPLEMENTS THAT HELP BLOOD-SUGAR PROBLEMS

Onions and garlic have been found to be helpful in addressing blood sugar problems. Eat them liberally, both in raw and cooked form, or take garlic supplements that are odorless

Additionally, ginger root, cinnamon, fenugreek seed, nutmeg, and bay leaf have all been found to help reduce the body's need for insulin. You might want to add a teaspoon or so of one of these to a morning protein shake.

SUPPLEMENTS TO AID IN MUSCLE HEALTH

Antioxidants are some of the best supplements you can take to aid in muscle health and the restoration of muscle tissues after exercise. Exercise not only impacts muscle tissue, of course. Every organ of the body is affected.

Antioxidants are a class of chemical compounds, many of which are vitamins, that attack free radicals, which cause cancer in the body. These free radicals are unstable molecules that are the result of an oxidizing process in the body. Think of the way an apple turns brown when it is exposed to oxygen. Something of that same process takes place to produce free radicals in the body. Just as the natural healthy structure of the apple is affected, so tissues of the body are impacted by free radicals. When free radicals are at work in the body, they can kill good cells, destroy enzymes, and produce toxins that disrupt cellular membrane functions.

Vigorous exercise increases the number of free radicals roaming the body.[19]

Most people aren't aware that the body has a natural antioxidant system. As exercise increases free radicals, the body increases its production of natural antioxidants. When a person takes antioxidants in supplement form, they boost the body's own production of antioxidants and at the same time combat free radicals on their own. A double benefit!

The most powerful antioxidants are vitamins C and E, pycnogenol, grapefruit seed extract, carotenes (such as beta-carotene and lycopene), selenium, and N-acetyl-cysteine (NAC). Make sure you take sufficient antioxidant supplements every day.

GLUCOSE-DISPOSAL AGENTS

The supplement described below helps shuttle glucose in the form of glycogen to muscle cells, rather than fat cells, and also helps the muscle cells to accept amino acids, protein, and creatine more readily. This supplement is used most commonly by athletes who are concerned with maintaining muscle strength and staying lean.

Alpha-lipoic Acid

Commonly called ALA, lipoic acid, or thioctic acid, this substance is not a new supplement. It has been subjected to a great deal of research and has been prescribed in Germany for a number of years for adult-onset diabetes. The recommended dosage for athletes is eight hundred milligrams a day, taken in two two-hundred-milligrams doses and one four-hundred-milligrams dose after a post-exercise recovery meal. ALA is considered a universal antioxidant because it is both fat and water soluble. It is probably the most potent glucose-disposal agent on the market.

SUPPLEMENTS TO ASSIST DIGESTION
AND HELP CURB APPETITE

Bromelain, papain, and pancreatin aid in the digestion of proteins, carbohydrates, and fats.

Spirulina (blue-green algae) is a natural food supplement that has substantial amounts of protein, essential fatty acids, vitamins, and minerals. It is very low in calories and helps curb the appetite. This is also true for other green foods.

SUPPLEMENTS THAT HELP WITH JOINT PAIN

A significant number of overweight people complain of joint pain. They often have bursitis, tendonitis, various types of arthritis, and other afflictions that cause aching knees, shoulders, and other joints. This pain can sometimes become a limiting factor for those who desire to pursue a fat-loss program when it comes to exercise.

Think low-impact. Walk, rather than jog. And if even walking is problematic, head for a swimming pool or an eliptical runner.

There are also two major things you can do nutritionally:

Eat Grays Lake Kosher Gelatin.

Choose unflavored Grays Lake, not the sugar-laden Jell-O nor the sugar-free Jell-O that is enhanced with sweeteners. Gelatin is made from animal collagen, which is an essential structural protein that forms an important part of bones, tendons, and connective tissues. It contains an exceptionally high content of two amino acids that play an important role in collagen formation in the body: proline and glycine. In fact, it would take forty-three grams of dried egg white, thirty-five grams of dried nonfat milk, or eight to nine grams of lean beef to equal the amount of proline in just ten grams of hydrolyzed gelatin.

My wife and I use Grays Lake kosher gelatin. It's by far the best we have ever found. We use two tablespoons daily in a protein shake.

Take flax oil regularly.

Elsewhere in this book, I have recommended that you take a daily dose of flaxseed oil. This oil helps reduce pain associated with any type of inflammatory condition, including joint problems. Have you ever stopped to consider that arthritis, bursitis, and tendonitis all end with "itis"? That's the suffix that indicates "inflammation." Arthritis is an inflammation of the cartilage at the end of joints. Bursitis is the inflammation of the small fluid-filled sacks called bursae that are located in the joints. Tendonitis is an inflammation of tendons. The Omega-3 fatty acids in flaxseed oil help form prostaglandins that reduce inflammation.

There are a number of products on the market today that include other nutrients that have been shown to help with joint pain. Look for these ingredients on the label: glucosamine, chondroitin sulfate, fish oils EPA/DHA, gamma-linoleic acid (GLA), vitamin E, fat-soluble vitamin C (ascorbyl palmitate), and manganese aspartate. Individually, these nutrients have only marginal effectiveness but when taken together in a "complex" formula, they appear to be very beneficial.

One product that I use on a regular basis for joint pain and inflammation is Arthrogen. It is a combination of niacinamide and N-acetylcysteine. It works extremely well for all types of chronic pain. Another product that is excellent is called Inflamix.

Remember always that the more you lose excess fat from the body, and the more you routinely exercise and build muscle, the more likely you are to experience a lessening, and perhaps a total disappearance, of joint problems, especially problems in the knee. I know of one man who had bariatric surgery (described later in this book) and lost forty pounds in two months. He was happy about his weight loss, his lowered blood pressure, and his physician's willingness to allow him to control his Type II diabetes with diet alone, but he was *overjoyed* with the fact that he could walk two miles and climb stairs without any pain in his knees!

SOME PRODUCTS YOU SHOULD *NOT* TAKE

This should go without saying but I'll say it anyway: Don't smoke or drink alcohol. Alcohol and smoking aren't good for a person at any age, and are especially harmful as a person increases in age. Many people smoke because they believe it curbs appetite. Nicotine does curb appetite, but so do many things that are good for you, which nicotine is not. Choose to follow the advice in this book and you'll probably find that your cravings for nicotine decrease as your health increases and your fat melts away!

There are three products that I feel I must tell you not to take, or to take with great caution.

1. L-Phenylalanine

Do not take L-Phenylalanine if you are taking an MAO inhibitor (antidepressants often have these). If you are not sure, ask your physician. Do not use it if you have cardiac arrhythmias, hypertension, the genetic disease PKU, psychosis, or existing pigmented malignant melanoma-type cancer, or if you have a violent temper.

Even small doses can cause permanent brain damage. As explained in an earlier chapter, L-Phenylalanine is one of the primary components of aspartame, the artificial sweetener. Never use this product.

2. Steroids

Do not take steroids to try to build up muscle mass in your body. Steroids do help muscles grow faster, but the results of steroid use can be devastating. Most steroid compounds are illegal—the buying, selling, and using of anabolic steroids are all crimes. Problems in the human body seem to range from severe acne to water retention, from the development of gynecomastia (build-up of breast tissue in the mammary glands of men) to premature hair loss. More serious health problems have also been implicated, including premature death. The risks just aren't worth any short-term results you might experience.

The fact is if you are hitting the weights hard and following a proper nutrition and supplementation program, you don't need steroids to build up your muscles.

3. Testosterone

You may have heard that you can take testosterone (through injection, use of patches, application of a gel or ointment, or by taking a pill) and reverse muscle loss. That's not necessarily so.

Testosterone can boost muscle mass and sexual drive. But it can also cause liver damage and accelerate the growth and proliferation of prostate cancer cells.

Testosterone had been linked to prostate tumors and a blocking of sperm production. It has also been linked to a reduction in HDL (good) cholesterol.

I encourage you to be very cautious in taking testosterone as a supplement. Testosterone-replacement therapy (which is to men what estrogen- and hormone-replacement therapy is to women) may have other negative side effects that we won't even know about until long-range scientific research studies are completed.

One of the interesting facts that has emerged from recent testosterone research is this: Middle-age men who maintain the body weight they had in their twenties may have no decline in testosterone levels at all, while overweight adult men of any age tend to have lower testosterone levels. Get your body-fat under control and you may have all the testosterone you can handle!

My testosterone and human growth hormone levels are still those of a twenty-two-year-old male. I'm forty-five years old and I feel great!

Testosterone patches, pills, or injections are available only on a prescription basis and can cost fifty dollars to one hundred dollars a month. In my opinion, that money is better spent on supplements that you know are beneficial to muscle health! If your health care professional suggests that you take either steroids or testosterone please get a second opinion and proceed with caution.

AT THE CUTTING EDGE: COMBINATIONS

Much research is being devoted today to experimenting with combinations of minerals, vitamins, and herbs. Combined nutrients often have a synergistic effect—in other words, the nutrients have multiplied benefits when put together, and a much higher benefit than if you took the nutrients separately. One such combination is zinc, glycine, and arginine. Each of these nutrients can contribute to healthy function in the body in a number of different and yet mutually supportive ways. When taken together, those benefits are *multiplied.*

Thermogenic Stacking

Many of the new combinations appearing on the market have to do with the body's thermodynamic (heat-producing) processes, helping to free fatty acids from body fat stores so they can be used for fuel. When these compounds are combined for even greater effectiveness, fat-loss experts call it *thermogenic stacking.*

Thermogenic stacks are best taken thirty to sixty minutes before exercise or a meal. They should not be taken after five o'clock at night because they may keep a person awake. Be sure to read the labels closely on these products and look for quality ingredients. Always buy such products only from a reputable distributor.

Remember, too, that these supplements work much better if you are exercising and eating properly. And please do not take these thermogenic products daily —only use them if you feel you have no other choice.

MORE HELP MAY BE ON THE HORIZON

A number of supplements are still being tested and seem to show promise right now for helping in the fight against fat. Choose to keep yourself informed as to the latest advancements in the war against obesity.

One supplement to watch is the human growth hormone (HGH), also called simply growth hormone (GH). Numerous research studies are showing that the genetically engineered human growth hormone is effective in causing weight reduction in animals. An inexpensive injection or capsule form of HGH for humans is still several years away and the long-term consequences of HGH use are unknown at present. Watch for more news on this.

Growth hormone, or somatotropin, is the most abundant hormone made by the pituitary. Cells in the pituitary produce GH and release it into the bloodstream, where it is absorbed by the liver and converted into various growth factors. Nearly every organ in the body is dependent on GH for proper growth and development.

As a person ages, GH levels decline. By the age of sixty, both men and women are only producing about half of the GH they did when they were twenty or thirty.

As the body ages, lean body mass starts to diminish as well, while fat stores increase. While this can't be blamed entirely on a decrease in GH levels, maintaining GH levels may be a key to keeping lean body mass at maximum levels.

GH has been used primarily by athletes who desire to keep their muscles bulked up. A benefit of GH, however, is not only muscle retention, but fat reduction. In some cases, the results have been startling. One French doctor, Thierry Hertoghe, reported that his patients on GH experienced between 23 and 30 percent reductions in the size of their "love handles." The fat melted away from undesirable areas (belly, thighs, back of arms) and seemed to be replaced in areas where it is desirable, such as the back of the hand and the hollow "dark-circle" and wrinkle areas of the face.

GH binds to the hormone receptors of fat cells, creating a host of enzymatic reactions that aid fat-burning. GH works also to prevent insulin from storing fat, and at the same time enhances the immune system by increase the size of the thymus, which is the leading producer of T-cells in the body.

A Swiss physician, Sam Baxas of the Baxamed Clinic, has been using GH to treat patients who have muscular sclerosis, lupus, Alzheimer's, Lou Gehrig's disease, and even AIDS. He's seen phenomenal results.[20]

The list of GH-associated benefits is long and growing longer. It appears to reverse heart disease by thickening the walls of weakened ventricles, improves LDL/HDL levels, prevents or reverses osteo-porosis, improves vision, increases brain power, improves or restores sexual erection, and possibly stimulates hair regrowth. Those who have received GH therapy report more rapid healing of fractures and wounds, a normalization of thyroid dysfunction, a normalizing of body temperature, and positive effects on male and female fertility.[21]

Wow. With all these seemingly positive effects, is there a down-side? Yes. Potential side effects come with an overdosing on GH and they are serious: diabetes, cancer, carpal tunnel syndrome, disfigur-ing cartilage growth. Taking more of a good thing is definitely not a good thing. Those who experience these negative results, however, have admitted to taking up to twenty times more than the standard dosage.

If you are interested in taking GH, work only with a physician who is well-read on the subject of GH therapy. In most cases, those who receive GH therapy do not receive the injections continuously. A "cycling" protocol seems most effective. You should also be aware that the drug remains very expensive. A full year of therapy could range from eight thousand dollars to eighteen thousand dollars. (Definitely avoid the urge to try to get this drug on the black market. Too many impure and totally bogus versions are out there.)

DEVELOP A RELATIONSHIP WITH THE EXPERTS

As you begin to explore various supplements, I encourage you to work with a licensed nutritional counselor. Ask questions. Listen to their advice about various products. You can learn a great deal about what to take, and what *not* to take, from a licensed nutritionist.

Always buy supplements from a reputable dealer. Make sure the products are clearly labeled as to their ingredients and recommended dosages.

If you have any doubt about taking a supplement, don't take it!

This is not an area where if a little is good, more is better. The body is delicately balanced, and that's by divine design!

Please, if you have any questions call my office. My highly-trained staff and I are there to help you. There is nothing more frustrating to me than to read an excellent book, want more information, and not have easy access to that information. That is why throughout this book I have referred to specific products and have encouraged you to call my toll-free number for mor information. I can only help you if you give me a chance. At least crop me a line so that I can add you to my mailing list for future updates.

18

THE REAL SCOOP
ON CELLULITE

Contrary to what many people think, cellulite is not a disease. Rather, it is a cosmetic disorder due to anatomical changes.

Cellulite is related to aging far more than to weight, although fat accumulation is involved. It is a skin condition that results in something called the *mattress phenomena*—a pitting, bulging, and deformation of the skin. The person with cellulite may feel a tightness or heaviness in the area affected, particularly the legs. The skin also feels tender if pinched, pressed upon, or vigorously massaged.

As most women probably suspect, 90 to 98 percent of cellulite cases occur in women.

WHAT CAUSES CELLULITE?

Cellulite is formed when excessive subcutaneous adipose tissue or a degeneration of subcutaneous connective tissue leads to the enlargement of fat chambers.

The word *cellulite* is actually a French word. It was adopted by the lay public in the United States before American physicians were educated in a condition that European physicians recognized for more than one hundred and fifty years.[1] The correct English word is actually be *cellulitis.* That word, however, refers to an inflammatory or infectious process involving the connective tissues under the skin. In cellulite there is no inflammatory or infectious process.

Researchers have suggested *dermo-panniculois deformans* or *adiposis edematosa* as correct terminology, but I think we can agree that those terms aren't likely to make it into the common American vocabulary. So, we have a word that isn't truly descriptive—except, of course, for those who have the condition!

Cellulite is found primarily on the thighs and the gluteal (buttocks) region. To a lesser extent, cellulite is found in the lower part of the abdomen, on the nape of the neck, and on the upper parts of the arms.

To really understand cellulite, you have to understand a little about the composition of skin. The outer layer of the skin is the dermis. The interior layers of the skin, not visible, are the subepidermal or subcutaneous tissues.

Subcutaneous tissue is composed of three layers of fat, with two planes of connective tissue between them. These tissues differ greatly in men and women. In women, the uppermost layer has large "standing fat-cell chambers," which are separated by dividing walls that appear arched if you take a side view of the fat cells. In men, this layer has a network of crisscrossing connective tissue walls. The connective tissue between the dermis and subcutaneous tissue is also thicker in men than women.[2]

You can actually see these differences in tissue structure by doing a pinch test. If you pinch the skin and subcutaneous tissue of the thighs of women, you tend to see something that looks like a "mattress." When you pinch the thigh skin of men, you'll find a folding or furrowing effect, but the skin does not bulge or pit.

As women age, the corium, a layer of the subcutaneous tissue, which is already thinner in women than in men, becomes increasingly thinner and looser.[3] This allows the fat cells to migrate into this layer. The connective tissue walls also become thinner, allowing the fat-cell chambers to enlarge excessively. As the connective tissue structures break down, a granular or buck-shot feeling develops in the area affected.

The "mattress phenomenon" comes about as a result of the alternating depressions and protrusions in the upper compartments of fat tissue. All the while, as the corium layer becomes thinner, lymphatic vessels of the upper corium layer become distended, and the number of subepidermal elastic fibers decreases.

The Four Stages of Cellulite

Cellulite tends to be classified in four stages:

Stage 0. This is the stage in which the skin on the thighs and buttocks has a smooth surface when a person is standing or lying. When the skin is pinched, it folds and furrows but does not pit or bulge. This is the normal stage of most men and slim women.

Stage 1. In this stage, the skin surface is smooth when a subject is standing or lying, but the pinch test clearly shows a mattress phenomenon. This is normal for most females. (If males experience this, there may be a deficiency of androgenic hormones.)

Stage 2. In this stage, the skin surface is smooth while the subject is lying, but when standing, the affected skin surface shows pitting, bulging, and deformity. This is common in women who are obese or past forty years of age.

Stage 3. The final stage is when the mattress phenomenon is apparent when a subject is lying or standing. It is very common after menopause and in obese women.

Although most women might consider Stage 0 to be their ideal goal, the best classification most can expect is Stage 1 simply because of the female anatomy. Don't expect ever to get rid of all cellulite. It's a fact of aging. Do try to remain at Stage 1!

PREVENTING CELLULITE

The best approach, as is true regarding most chronic diseases as well as cosmetic conditions, is prevention. Since the size and number of fat cells in any person is largely determined by the person's mother and her prenatal nutrition, many people have a significant predisposition toward cellulite.

Prevention begins by maintaining a slim subcutaneous fat layer. Regular exercise and a normal body weight throughout life are key. Slim women and female athletes have little or no cellulite.

The primary treatment of cellulite is weight reduction coupled with exercise. The weight reduction should be gradual, especially in women older than forty. *A rapid loss of weight in individuals whose skin and connective tissues are already undergoing changes from aging will often make the mattress phenomenon more obvious.*

Massage is very beneficial, particularly self-administered massage with the hand or a brush. The physical and mechanical effects of massage improve the circulation of blood and lymph. The direction of the massage should always be from the periphery of the area toward the heart.

There are a number of cosmetic formulas on the market that claim to be effective in curing cellulite. The majority of these formulas, however, have no scientific basis. Long-term double-blind research studies of some of the more popular cellulite treatments have shown that they are no more effective than a placebo.[4] There are *botanical* compounds, however, that have confirmed effects in treating cellulite.

HERBAL TREATMENTS FOR CELLULITE

If cellulite is caused by enlarged subcutaneous fat layers and weakening connective tissue bonds, then the solution to cellulite is fairly clear. Reverse those two trends! *Reduce* subcutaneous fat—that's what fat-loss is all about. *Strengthen* the connective tissue bonds

It only makes sense that herbal medicines that strengthen connective tissue would be beneficial. The reduction of fat requires adopting the complete program presented in this book. You can't expect herbs to take care of that part of the process. A comprehensive herbal treatment for cellulite involves both oral and topical medicines that enhance connective tissue structures.

Four main herbal products have been shown to be beneficial:

Centella Asiatica

Centella asiatica, an extract of centella, has been shown in clinical studies to be an impressive treatment for cellulite as well as varicose veins.[5] It works primarily by normalizing the metabolism of connective tissues and by helping to build normal connective tissue. This compound also improves blood flow through affected areas.

Escin

Escin is a compound isolated from the seeds of the horsechestnut. It has anti-inflammatory and anti-edema properties related to the capillaries and it has been shown to help those with varicose veins and thrombophlebitis.[6] In the treatment of cellulite, escin can be taken orally or applied topically as an escin-cholesterol complex. It is not only beneficial for cellulite, but also for the treatment of bruises.

Bladderwrack

Bladderwrack (also known as *Fucus vesiculosus*) is a seaweed that has been used in the treatment of obesity since the seventh century. It has a high iodine content that seems to stimulate thyroid function if taken orally. As a topical treatment, it has been effective in soothing, softening, and toning the skin.[7]

Cola Herb

Cola herb is a rich source of caffeine and related compounds. This compound is administered topically in the treatment of cellulite.

Let me reinforce the idea that these herbal compounds cannot help you reduce the fat layers in subcutaneous tissue. They help strengthen connective tissue bonds. Losing fat is the real heart of remedying cellulite.

For most women, that's all the more reason to work hard for maximum fat loss!

19

A PLEA FOR
OUR CHILDREN

Not only are we fatter as adults, but our children and teens are fatter. We are experiencing a national epidemic of obesity among our young.

The proportion of overweight children jumped from 5 percent in 1964 to nearly 13 percent in 1994, the most recent year on record. If that trend has continued—and many believe it has actually accelerated—one child in three is now either overweight or at risk of becoming obese.

No race or class has been spared when it comes to childhood obesity. And, it seems, no child is too young to experience real problems related to obesity.

Overweight children are now showing up in clinics across our nation with problems such as fatty liver (a precursor to cirrhosis) and sleep apnea (a condition in which excess flesh around the throat blocks the airway causing snoring, fitful sleep and a chronic lack of oxygen that can damage the heart and lungs). Several years ago, I attended a health and preventive medicine seminar in Colorado. I met a pediatrician there who was an expert on childhood disease and obesity. He told me that he had never examined an older teenager who did not already have arterial plaquing, a precursor to heart disease and stroke. One of his primary dietary recommendations for these children is: *No pizza!*

Why are our children increasingly obese? Even rarely when children are genetically predisposed to being overweight, lifestyle factors are what trigger that predisposition into obesity. Lifestyle factors involve primarily two things: how a child eats and how a child exercises.

The time to maintain a lean weight is all of one's life, starting in the child and teen years. The time to exercise is all of one's life.

THE TERRIBLE CONSEQUENCES OF OBESITY IN CHILDREN

Type II diabetes is turning up in overweight kids. In times past, Type II diabetes rarely occurred until age forty. Now, about a third of pediatric patients are Type II. This type of diabetes has the potential for damaging blood vessels within a decade, and setting up a child for later kidney failure, blindness, amputations, heart attacks, and strokes.

Sadly, many children are not being screened for diabetes, although more and more physicians are calling for chronically overweight kids to be tested early and treated vigorously.

In a Head Start research study involving New York City preschoolers, a researcher from Columbia University found that children as young as three and four years of age were showing signs of elevated blood pressure and cholesterol.

Dr. William Dietz of the Centers for Disease Control and Prevention has said, "There's a lag between the development of obesity and the chronic diseases associated with it. We're in that trough right now. Very soon we'll see the rate of cardiovascular disease among teenagers rising."[1]

Most people are not aware that one out of every four teenagers presently carries enough excess weight to put him or her at high risk of heart attack, stroke, cancer, gout, and other serious health problems later in life . . . and that's regardless of whether the individual slims down as an adult.

TEACH YOUR CHILD HOW TO EAT

Many parents assume that when they teach their children how to manipulate a spoon, a fork, and a knife that they have taught their children how to eat. No! They have taught their children how to get food from a plate to the mouth in a polite manner. Teaching your child how to eat involves teaching your child what to stick a knife, fork, and spoon into!

A *New England Journal of Medicine* study in September 1997 reported that if parent's are obese, there is more than double the chance that their children will become obese as adults. Genetics plays some role, but the far greater likelihood is that children are imitating their parents' eating and exercise habits. We each tend to eat what our parents taught us to eat, and to exercise in the same way they did—for most fat people, that means no exercise at all!

Too often unhealthy school lunches and readily available vending machines with high-fat snacks and diet sodas are part of the equation for children. The constant temptation is there for kids: McDonald's and other fast food chains compete for their dollars. Candy and sodas are a mainstay.

Three Specific Things to Teach Your Child

There are three specific and very beneficial things you can teach your children from their earliest years.

1. Teach your child which foods to eat and which to avoid. Strictly limit the consumption of sweets, high fat dairy products, and other high-fat foods. Offer healthy alternatives as snack food. I recently saw a television show on extremes. One of the stories featured a house cat that weighed nearly fifty pounds. The commentator said the cat's

favorite food was biscuits. This came as no surprise. Be sure to add bread to your list of foods that are off limits.

2. Teach your child how to "just say no" to high-calorie, high-fat, high-sugar snacks and foods offered to them by insisting peers. Give them coping mechanisms for saying no firmly but politely. Give them factual information to support your reasons for desiring them to stay away from foods that can lead to obesity.

3. Teach your child how to make a protein shake. Even fairly young children can learn how to put ingredients—protein powder, fruit, ice cubes—into a blender, put on the lid, and push a button. There's no excuse for sending your child off to school without proper nutrients. Studies have shown that children who eat breakfast do better in school. They have also shown that protein eaten in the morning has beneficial effects well into early afternoon. A protein shake can really give your child an "edge" in learning.

My twelve-year-old and my eighteen-month-old both share my protein shake daily. If my eighteen-month-old loves the shake and gets upset if he doesn't get it quickly enough, an adult should have no excuse! (The recipe for this shake is in the *Maximum Fat Loss Workbook*.)

ENCOURAGE YOUR CHILD TO BE ACTIVE

Don't raise a couch potato. Get your children involved in physical activities that are fun for them. It may be karate, softball, soccer, gymnastics, or aerobic dance classes.

I recently heard about a family that has four children who are very physically active, but they don't necessarily enjoy the same sports. The older boy is big into baseball, the older girl is a junior lifeguard and loves swimming, the younger girl takes tennis lessons four days a week because she loves the game so much, and the younger boy is happiest when a basketball is in his hands. One thing I know is that the parents of these children are also active taking them to various lessons, practices, games, and matches! The children are active in sports they truly enjoy, and as a result, they are likely to remain active in those sports for much longer.

Take time to discover what your child enjoys doing, not necessarily what you wish your child would enjoy. In this particular family, Dad was a college football player and Mom enjoyed equestrian sports. Neither Mom nor Dad has insisted that their children follow in their footsteps, and their children are happier in the wake of the parents' wise decision to let their children dictate their sports of choice.

Many children shy away from sports because they have felt rejected by teammates or have concluded that they "just aren't good at sports." Every child can do something well. And if your child is succeeding at an activity, he will want to do it more often.

Rather than allow your child to watch TV or play video games hour after hour, insist that your child go outside to play. If your outdoor neighborhood isn't safe, get your child into a neighborhood gym. Do your utmost to keep your child physically active.

Keep in mind that physical activity need not be in competitive sports or injury-prone team sports. Get your child involved in activities such as a Christian karate class, an aerobics dance class, a noncompetitive swimming program, golf lessons (and let them walk the course without the benefit of a golf cart), or other non-team athletic activities. My wife and my older son both have their black belts! I tease my wife by telling her that I am uncomfortable around her when she is angry. But all kidding aside, I am a lot more comfortable knowing that she is safe when she is out shopping by herself.

Your children need to be involved in three types of exercise:

Cardiovascular

Walk or cycle with your child. Walking regularly with your child can become a good time for talking as well!

Weight-training

Begin this training lightly after your child is about eleven or twelve years old. Younger children can be encouraged to do a few dips, push-ups, and bench presses with high repetitions and low weights. My twelve-year-old works out with me daily.

Flexibility

Even very young children can learn to do simple stretching exercises. After walking with your child or teen, take time to stretch!

It's time to restore physical education to schools.

I find it troublesome that most parents believe their children need to be plugged into computers at school, while at the same time, these parents seem quite willing for physical education classes to go by the wayside. The facts are clear—youngsters and teens who don't get enough exercise are at greater risk for obesity, diabetes, cancer, and heart disease. Youngsters who don't spend an extra half hour at a computer? That's hardly a career-breaking or an education-smashing factor!

In one study involving 17,700 middle school and high school students, researchers found that those who had a physical-education class five times a week were more than twice as likely to be highly active in their nonschool hours. Those who didn't have physical education classes tended to spend their out-of-school time watching television or videos and playing video or computer games. Sadly, only one-fifth of the youngsters surveyed were enrolled in a physical education class, and only 15 percent had a physical-education class five times a week.

Fewer than half of our nation's schools offer physical education. Virginia is the only state that still mandates recess as part of the daily routine.

Cynics predict that as a nation we'll get serious about childhood obesity about twenty years from now, when today's children are hobbled by arteriosclerosis and end-stage renal disease. Not being a cynic, my approach is this: Let's do something *now!*

FAT IMPACTS YOUR CHILD'S SELF-ESTEEM

A young man I know named Doug went to live with his father after his parents separated. Dad didn't know much about cooking so the two of them ate a tremendous amount of pizza—probably five nights out of seven they had pizza for dinner. Both of them ballooned into obesity.

The more Doug gained, the more he lost—self-esteem, that is. He lost some of his socialization skills and his circle of friends diminished. His grades declined. Dad tried to place the blame for his poor school performance on the marital separation. That may have been partly at fault. What Dad failed to see was that his son was also very self-conscious about his weight gain and no longer wanted to go to the apartment-complex swimming pool or hang out with his friends at the beach.

When Doug and his dad started working out together, cut out the pizza, and made a few other fat-loss changes in their lives, not only did Doug lose weight but his self-esteem rose. So did his grades and his sociability.

Weight and self-esteem are vitally linked in children. What a child weighs is directly linked to how a child perceives himself and defines his self-identity.

Give Your Child a Challenge.

Every child wants to look good, feel good, and feel as if he can accomplish physical challenges—including weight loss and exercise challenges. In overcoming an obstacle or in accomplishing a physical feat, children grow in self-esteem.

I saw that clearly just a few weeks ago in a young man I'll call Joe.

I volunteered to chaperone a group of youth from my church to Mount LeConte. The hike up one side is about five and a half miles, for a total hike of eleven miles up and back. Several of the kids who hiked with me, including my son Austin, were trained athletes or were in good physical shape. Also in our party was Joe, a young boy about ten years old who was about fifty pounds overweight.

I knew it would be very difficult for Joe to do an eleven-mile hike in the shape he was in. I immediately set myself toward encouraging him every step of the way. We stopped often for him to catch his breath, and at each stop, I told him how great he was doing. We made the entire experience a very positive one for him and before the day was over, he had completed the entire eleven-mile trek.

At the base of the mountain, I stood back and looked at this boy, and let me tell you he couldn't have been standing any taller or prouder. Not only that, but Joe began to follow a health plan I shared with him on the drive home. A month after he began the plan, he had lost five pounds. He was determined to take charge of his own health and fat loss. What a kid!

A Classic Case Study in Childhood Obesity

We have a young friend who is something of a classic case study when it comes to the negative consequences of childhood obesity—consequences not necessarily on health but on the *life* of a child.

Our friend was very healthy as a child until he was about eight years old. Then his parents eliminated all sports activities from his life and suggested that he focus all of his attention on his computer and academic endeavors. I think they saw a lack of sports as a means of keeping him free of injury, and also lowering any stress that might be associated with competition. It must also be noted that they were not the type of parents who would take the time to drive him around to these activities. At the same time, they saw computers as the wave of the future and hoped that by fueling his interest in computers he would do better in school and have a jump on his classmates when it came time for college and career.

This boy became a computer nerd and led a sedentary life. Every time we visited this family—which was about once a year—I was shocked to see how much weight he had gained since our previous visit. I finally said something to his parents.

Their response was basically this: Our son's weight is none of your business, and besides, it really isn't a problem. He will grow out of this "baby fat" as he gets into his teen years.

The next visit to our house, the family went with us to water ski. At age thirteen, this boy now weighed about two hundred pounds. He couldn't get up on the skis that day and was very upset at his failure. Even though I had been told to back off, I approached his parents again to talk to them about their son's weight. This time I offered to give them some of my materials so that they might help him. The parents turned a deaf ear and actually became angry.

The next year this young man weighed about two hundred and forty pounds. I knew his self-esteem had to be taking a serious hit. He began hanging out with a group of kids who were also overweight and were misfits at his school. As a means of gaining popularity, this teenage boy turned to what I believe was using and then selling drugs. He led a clandestine lifestyle, lying to his parents all the while.

By the time he went to college, he weighed close to three hundred pounds. Several years later, I had an opportunity to visit with him and I was shocked. He had pierced and tattooed just about every part of his body that could be pierced or tattooed, and he was sporting a green and orange Mohawk haircut. He had also lost a great deal of weight. How? I believe it was through excessive use of dangerous and illegal drugs.

A year later, he had lost over a hundred pounds and his flesh was yellow-orange from what I suspected to be all the damage he had done to his liver through drug use.

I decided that talking to his parents was no longer the way to go and I went to this young man directly. I said, "Listen, here's the deal. I don't care how many nipple and nose rings you have. The only thing I'm concerned about is that you don't use drugs."

He got really quiet and grew pale. I don't think he had any idea that any adult in his life suspected he was using drugs. I went on. "You really think you're going to get into graduate school someday as you tell me you hope to do, but I can tell you that you aren't going to be admitted to a graduate program with all of these piercings and your body looking like it does. I promise you they simply won't take you seriously, regardless of your grades or test scores."

Right after I spoke to him, he began to change his attitude. He dealt with his hair and the piercings, and I hope he stopped any illegal drug use in which he may have been involved.

Here's what I think happened to this young man. I think most of his rebellious actions—the piercings, hairstyle, and even the substance abuse—stemmed from the very low self-esteem he experienced primarily because he was obese and didn't know how to lose his excess body fat.

Excess fat is not beautiful. It is not appealing—not to the objective person who is viewing it and not to the person who is carrying it on his or her own body. When we see ourselves as less than what we can be—physically, emotionally, socially, intellectually, and even spiritually—we adopt a negative attitude toward ourselves. Our self-esteem—perhaps you want to call it self-value or self-worth—takes a hit. If you don't deal with the root cause of what is creating that less-than-positive image, you will try to justify the negatives in your life, which only reinforces and expands them. A vicious cycle sets in.

Now I am not at all advocating that a person can or should strive to be perfect in every area of life. That's not possible and it should never be a goal.

What is realistic—and what I do advocate strongly—is that every person work hard to develop and function at the fullness of his or her potential. That potential is physical as well as intellectual, emotional, relational, and spiritual. We have been given bodies to use, not abuse. We have been given a physical self to take care of, not to ignore. We have been given intelligence to apply toward our own physical health and we must choose to build ourselves up to the best health possible, not choose to tear ourselves down to the point where we become disheartened about ourselves.

HOW TO HELP YOUR CHILD

There are four very specific things you as a parent can do to help your child, starting today.

First, decide that you will never again wink at a weight gain or at bad eating habits, saying, "It doesn't matter." It *does* matter. It matters a great deal in your child's short-term and long-term health.

At the same time, never make fun of overweight people to your children. Being overweight is no laughing matter. Overweight people have feelings. They are not a joke. This is a very serious condition.

Second, help your child to adopt a healthful way of eating. That's a far better approach than talking to your children about going on a diet. Children who become extremely diet-conscious at an early age are often being set up for eating disorders. They assume that their parents don't like the way they look and therefore don't like who they are. Rather, take the approach, "I love you and we're both going to start eating in a way that will give us both the best quality of life we can hope to experience!"

Third, *lavish huge amounts of unconditional love* on your child. Accept your child for who he or she is, regardless of what he or she weighs. Unconditional love is the great preventive medicine for anorexia and bulimia and other eating disorders.

Fourth, model for your child the behaviors that you want your child to have. Exercise with your child. Eat nutritious meals and drink nutrious protein shakes with your child. Order nutritious meals when you are eating out with your child. Manifest the behaviors that you want your child to adopt as a life pattern.

The Bible even admonishes parents to raise up their children to know what is good and bad. That includes knowing what is good and bad for the human body. To train your child goes beyond mere talking. It means to require certain behaviors and to instill certain habits through repetition.

The best thing you can do for your child's health—both physical and emotional—is to train your child to eat and exercise in such a way that he never becomes fat in the first place! That's far better than having to train your child later in how to lose fat. My wife has written an excellent cookbook entitled, *Train Up Your Children in the Way They Should Eat.* It describes healthy eating habits from infancy through the teenage years.

20

SURGICAL OPTIONS FOR
CUTTING FAT

One of the most popular procedures today for removing fat deposits from the body is liposuction. We routinely see Hollywood stars who claim benefits from fat removed from their abdomens, buttocks, love handles, and the inner part of the upper legs—or so the liposuction providers declare in their commercials and infomercials.

The reality is this: Liposuction doesn't work for *most* people as a weight-loss remedy.

If you are going to have liposuction surgery, recognize two things. First, you are going to have *surgery*, with all of the attendant risk factors associated with any surgery. Second, make certain that your surgeon is board-certified in his specialty, make sure you have a legitimate board-certified cosmetic surgeon do the procedure. I recently heard about a dentist—yes, a dentist—who attended a twelve-hour weekend seminar on liposuction and then began doing the procedure. That certainly isn't a man I'm going to trust to touch any part of my body, much less perform liposuction surgery on me.

A friend of mine, seeking anonymity and confidentiality, recently drove a couple hours away from his home town to have liposuction surgery. He went to a medical doctor who ran large ads claiming to be a liposurgeon specialist. He performed the surgery right in his office, all of which sounded appealing to my friend.

The first liposurgery session was a disaster. The physician left sizable pockets of stored fat in various places, causing lumps all over his body, and leaving seventeen incisions and resulting scars on his hips, back, and abdomen. The doctor's statement to my friend was, "You can come back for 'touch-ups' if we've missed anything." The touch-ups, of course, were going to be at a very high fee. If a physician tells you touch-ups cost anything, run away, don't walk! (By the way, during the surgery the doctor had one of his friends come into the make-shift surgery suite, and then his wife joined them along with the family's dog! Unbelievable!)

My friend—out of desperation—went back to this man for touch-ups of the lumps, and this time the physician failed to anesthetize him properly. He was in such horrible pain that he insisted that the surgery be stopped before it was completed. The result for him was scars, lumps, and pain that haunt him to this day. He still has nightmares about these procedures.

And not only nightmares, the fat has moved to other parts of his body!

Nobody had explained to my friend that liposurgery not only removes fat, it removes the fat-storing cells along with the fat. That means if an individual regains the fat weight after this procedure has been performed, the body will look for another place to store the fat. Not finding the usual cells for storing fat, it will look for whatever cells it can find for fat storage.

My friend later learned that this physician had acquired his liposurgery skills in a weekend seminar class. Furthermore, he had no medical malpractice insurance for doing this procedure and did not have hospital-admitting privileges to any of the local hospitals. His medical school had even gone out of business. In other words, if something went wrong with a surgery in his office, he couldn't even get his victim the necessary medical assistance in a timely manner. In sum, he was not a board-certified cosmetic surgeon and when it came to plastic surgery procedures, he was for all practical purposes untrained.

Apart from checking to see that a doctor doing lipo-surgery is board-certified plastic surgeon, watch for two other things:

1. If a liposurgeon tells you that you need to lose fifty pounds before you have the procedure, you aren't a candidate for the procedure! That person is only after your money and may actually be endangering your health by insisting on such a weight loss before the procedure.

2. Make sure the liposurgeon works with local anesthesia, not a general anesthesia. General anesthesia has risk factors that are far too high.

Now I am not dismissing all liposurgery. There can be some benefits to this, especially in cases where stored fat pockets may be causing pressure on certain nerves or impacting the pain associated with severe scoliosis. It also can be useful if fat pockets are localized and haven't responded to exercise and proper eating. You need to make certain, however, that you adhere to these three guidelines:

1. Only pursue liposuction after making a very diligent effort at exercising. Give yourself several months of concerted exercise before you conclude that a fat pocket isn't going away.

2. Do not lose large amounts of weight prior to having this procedure.

3. Do not gain back any weight after the procedure. All you will do is chase the body fat around your body. If you are a woman with a stomach-fat problem, you may have liposuction only to acquire heavy upper arms and legs. If you are a man with love handles, you may have liposuction only to acquire a lumpy chest or fat pockets on your upper back. Of even greater consequence, those who have had major repeated lipo-surgery procedures can even get to the point where the body will seek to store excess fat around the vital organs.

BARIATRIC SURGERY AS AN OPTION

For a very tiny minority, bariatric surgery may be an option. This is legitimate surgery, and it does work for most of the people who have it.

Bariatric surgery is one of the major fat-fighting methods available today. Some have called this surgery the "unspoken option" in weight loss. It is a solution, however, that many people find intriguing.

Bariatric surgery is the method that pop singer Carly Wilson opted to take and that she made popular through an Internet-broadcast surgery a couple of years ago. Let me give you some basic information about this procedure so you can consider it carefully as a possible option.

In the first place, bariatric surgery is only for those who are classified as *clinically severely obese* or *morbidly obese.* In most cases, those who are morbidly obese have or will have severe health problems resulting from their obesity.

In an earlier section, we discussed briefly the obesity classification of *morbidly obese,* based upon ideal body weight (IBW) and Body Mass Index (BMI). The morbidly obese are those who usually weight more than one hundred pounds above their ideal body weight with a BMI higher than 40. Approximately 1.4 million people fall into this category. For them, bariatric surgery may be an option.

Those who are clinically, severely obese often have a number of contributing causes for their obesity: heredity, environment, culture, psychological, and socioeconomic. Their obesity is not always a disorder of willpower. For the morbidly obese person, bariatric surgery helps in virtually all of these areas.

Again, let me reinforce the idea that Bariatric surgery is not cosmetic surgery. It is a surgery intended to help the severely obese patient and lies squarely in the field of General Surgery. It has however been endorsed by the National Institute of Health Consensus Conference.

How Bariatric Surgery Works

To understand this surgical procedure, we need to review a little anatomy.

Normally when we chew and swallow food, the food moves down the esophagus to the stomach, where strong acid begins to digest it. The stomach can hold about three pints of food at any given time. The food then moves to the duodenum, the first section of the small intestine. There, bile and pancreatic juices speed up the digestive process. The duodenum is also where calcium and iron are absorbed into the system.

Beyond the duodenum, the body has nearly twenty feet of small intestine, and that is where the rest of the food's calories and nutrients are absorbed. Those particles that cannot be digested in the small intestine are stored in the large intestine until they are eliminated.

Bariatric surgery grew out of surgical procedures that were performed to treat severe gastric ulcers, especially surgeries that removed large portions of the stomach or small intestine. Surgeons discovered that those who had these ulcer surgeries lost weight after surgery.

One of the first bypass operations was performed in 1954 and by the 1960s, intestinal bypass operations were routinely used for treating severe obesity. This type of operation produced weight loss largely by malabsorption. The problem was that it robbed the body of necessary nutrients and caused unpredictable side effects. This original form of intestinal bypass is no longer used.

Surgeons today use procedures that produce weight loss by limiting the amount of food the stomach can hold and use a modified bypass that somewhat limits the absorption of nutrients and calories. There are two ways these surgical procedures work:

1. *Restrictive Surgery.* In this type of surgery, food intake is restricted by creating a small pouch at the top of the stomach where the food enters it from the esophagus. This pouch initially holds about one ounce of food and expands to about two to three ounces over time. The pouch has a lower outlet with a diameter of about a

quarter of an inch. This small outlet delays the emptying of food and causes a feeling of fullness. A person who eats too much or too fast will quickly become full, and if they persist, vomiting occurs.

To restrict the size of the stomach, a "banding" procedure is used. Gastric Banding (GB) and Vertical Banded Gastroplasty (VGB) are the common operations. There are modifications, such as silicone ring vertical gastroplasty (SRVG) and adjustable silicone gastric banding (ASGB).

In GB, the band is placed around the stomach near the upper end. This may be done through laparoscopy or open-abdomen surgery. VBG is the most frequently used procedure—both a band and staples are used to create the small stomach pouch.

2. *Stomach Bypass Surgery.* The two most common bypass operations first create a small stomach pouch and then bypass portions of the small intestines. These operations are called Roux-en-Y (RGB) and Biliopancreatic Diversion (BPD). RGB is the most common. In this surgery, a small pouch is created by stapling—this pouch has about one ounce in capacity. The small intestine is cut about eighteen inches below the stomach and a Y-shaped section of the small intestine is attached to the pouch allowing the food to bypass the duodenum. The food enters the second part of the small bowel within about ten minutes after a meal is consumed.

In BPD a portion of the stomach is removed and the final segment of the small intestine is attached to the small stomach pouch, bypassing the duodenum and upper intestine. (BPD is similar to the old intestinal bypass of the 1970s.) This procedure makes it difficult for the body to absorb nutrients, minerals, and vitamins. Patients who have BPD often suffer numerous deficiencies along with diarrhea.) I do not recommend this approach.

What Might You Expect?

First, bariatric surgery patients have a feeling of satisfaction after eating a very small amount of food. They do not have the cravings or sense of starvation that other dieters sometimes feel. They also have long-term proven success rates. Patients who have this surgery usually continue to lose weight for eighteen to twenty-four months after surgery. A fourteen-year follow-up study of six hundred patients (with a 96 percent follow-up rate), reported weight losses in the 50 percentile. This means that, depending upon the procedure used, a patient is likely to lose 50 to 75 percent of excess body weight and keep it off.

Not only that, but most bariatric patients experience a certain euphoria during the months after their surgery, partly because they are not hungry and their weight is coming off so quickly. They also are feeling better in general—other problems associated with their obesity begin to disappear. One bariatric surgery center followed 157 patients and reported more than 95 percent relief and resolution of these medical conditions that were associated or impacted by their obesity: hypertension, dyslipidemia, diabetes mellitus, cholelithiasis, psychosocial impairment, obstructive sleep apnea, hypoventilation syndrome, degenerative arthritis, hypertrophic cardiomyopathy, hernias, urinary stress incontinence, infertility, gastro-esophageal reflux, lower extremity venous statis disease, blood clots, increased risk of certain cancers, increased risk of stroke, and socioeconomic impairment. Very rarely can one type of surgery yield so many positive results for a patient!

Not Without Risk

Bariatric surgery is *surgery*, and all surgery has risk factors. Certainly the person who brings one hundred to two hundred excess pounds to the operating table brings even more risk to the surgery suite. The risk of dying from gastric bypass surgery is far lower, however, than that of dying from complications related to obesity. More than 91 percent of those who have Bariatric surgery have no postoperative complications.

The fact is an estimated three hundred thousand Americans die as a direct result of obesity each year. The National Bariatric Surgery

Registry reported that within forty days of this kind of surgery, only .13 percent of the patients surveyed died. (In this particular study, that means only ten people out of 7,415.)

An ongoing Swedish obesity study is following the progress of two thousand obese men and women who were randomly assigned to either gastric resection surgery or to drug and diet therapy. To date, only three people have died as a result of surgery, compared to twenty-seven people who were in the nonsurgical group.[1]

In simple terms, the risks for this surgery are there, but in some cases there is no other alternative.

Costs and Referral

If you are considering this type of surgery, you need to have some specifics. The cost can range from ten thousand to twenty thousand dollars. There are about fifteen thousand of these operations done every year in the United States. If you do not know a Bariatric surgeon in your area, you may contact the American Society for Bariatric Surgery at 6717 N.W. 11th Place, Suite C, Gainesville, FL 32605. You can check out their Internet site at http://www.asbs.org.

In some cases, insurance will cover this surgery. There are several things you can do to help get a positive response from your insurance company. First, have your surgeon write a letter that clearly demonstrates the medical necessity of the surgery. They should cite your long battle with obesity, your current weight, diet history and failures, BMI, risk and comorbid conditions. Insurance companies rarely authorize a surgery unless a person has a BMI of 35 or higher and two comorbid conditions. It will also be helpful to have a letter from other practitioners who may know you as a patient, such as your internist, cardiologist, pulmonary specialist, or psychiatrist. Provide as much documentation as possible.

If you are turned down by your insurance company, you may want to contact the Obesity Law Center at 3160 Camino Del Rio South,

Suite 312, San Diego, CA 92108. They also have an Internet site: http://www.obesitylaw.com.

One of the best Internet sites related to obesity surgery is Owen's Links at http://homepages.ihug.co.nz/ olwen/ocwlnkws.htm.
If you want to join an on-line support group for patients thinking about this surgery or people who have had this surgery, contact http://www.onelist.com/subscribe.cgi/ossg. (Be forewarned, however—you are likely to receive one to two hundred messages a day!)

Another site that specializes who have had RGB is http://www.onelist.com (surgical weight loss support group).

DO WHAT YOU CAN FIRST

Keep in mind that both liposuction and bariatric surgery require a significant change in life habits after they are done. They are not a cure-all that requires no ongoing effort from you—to the contrary! They require extreme diligence in keeping fat from reentering the body and keeping too much food from being put back into the digestive tract. These surgeries are not a substitute for discipline.

Consider surgery your absolute last resort in fat loss. It is an option for some. For the vast majority of people, the twelve keys offered in this book will deal with fat in an effective way, and in a way that can become a life habit. Give your diligent best to pursuing all twelve keys in this book. Then, and only then, look at your surgical options.

21

CHOOSE TO BE LEAN
AND FIT ALL YOUR LIFE

Maximum fat loss is not just about short-term results. It is about developing a program that will help you reach your goal and stay there the rest of your life!

Long-term weight-loss success tends to be measured by a very simple standard: Reach your goal weight and stay there for a year. I believe in a longer standard: Stay lean always!

Maintaining fat loss is a lifetime pursuit for me. I grew a great many fat cells as a child and fat cells never leave the human body. They are always lying there in something of a flattened dormant state just waiting to be filled up again. My challenge for the rest of my days is to maintain control over those fat cells and to refuse to allow any fat to get back into them.

A DAILY CHALLENGE

A lean body is a daily challenge. It is something that must be sought and diligently pursued every day, day in and day out, week in and week out.

Choose to encourage yourself daily that you can and will do what it takes to remain healthy.

This is the day the Lord has made. I will rejoice and be glad in it!

Make that your attitude every day. It doesn't matter if the sun is shining or if the boss is in a good mood or if the traffic is smooth-flowing. You are the one who determines your attitude toward the circumstances around you.

I have met many people through the years who become devastated if they "fall off the wagon" of their fat-loss program they abandon their fat loss goals as hopelessly beyond their reach and they refuse to begin again with the next meal to monitor their food intake.

Don't let that happen to you. Choose to rejoice in your life. If you make a mistake at one meal, or even for one entire day, make a decision the next morning that "today is a new day" and begin again.

Trust God to help you with the dawn of each new day to make the choices that will benefit your health and keep you moving forward toward your fat-loss goals.

The average person thinks fifty thousand thoughts a day. If a significant number of those thoughts are ones that you turn negatively toward yourself—mentally berating yourself for ineptness or if you are punishing yourself for your set-backs—you will become discouraged.

I once met a woman named Leigh who beat herself up mentally every time she ate something that she knew she shouldn't eat. Every time she came to see me, she spent at least fifteen minutes confessing all the failures of the previous two weeks. She had mentally rehearsed each failure countless times. Her failures were at the forefront of her thinking. What Leigh didn't realize was that she was programming her own mind and attitude for future failures! She was embedding deep in her own thought processes the message, *I am a failure at this. I am a failure at this. I am a failure at this.*

You can't brainwash yourself with failure messages continually and then automatically make success choices!

Rather than focus on one meal that is a failure, focus on the meals that were good ones. Say to yourself, *Today was an 80 percent successful day. Tomorrow I'm going for a 100 percent.*

Choose to correct a slip at the very next meal in your life. As soon as you recognize you have made a mistake in what you have chosen to eat, how much you have eaten, or the way you have prepared certain foods . . . start anticipating your success at the next meal. Erase the past from your memory bank and consider the next meal to be "the first meal of the rest of your life."

If you experience a slip in your fat-loss program, make a decision that you are going to get over it. One slip-up is just that: one slip-up. Get right back into the saddle of good eating and good exercise.

Rehearse Your Resolve

Take a few minutes at the start of each day to recharge your resolve concerning your fat-loss program. I suggest that just before you drink that first morning protein drink or eat breakfast you sit down in a comfortable chair and spend three minutes just relaxing your body. Concentrate on a complete slackening of the muscles of your legs, pelvis, abdomen, arms, shoulders, and neck—in that order. Think through some of the positive statements that you have written down or established as goals or motivational triggers to help you stay on a fat-loss program.

Close your eyes and visualize yourself as having an abundance of physical energy, being lean and fit and healthy, and having good mental, emotional, and spiritual vitality for doing all that lies ahead for you.

Does this sound too simplistic? Try it for a week and I think you'll be amazed at what this three minutes in a morning can do to build new mental habits to go along with your fat-loss program.

GETTING OFF A PLATEAU

There are two important stages of a fat-loss program. The first is the *getting started* stage.

The second stage in a fat-loss program can actually occur a number of times before you reach your goal. It is the I'm-not-progressing-fast-enough stage. This stage usually occurs when you feel you have hit a plateau in your fat loss—a time when the scales just don't budge.

Both of these stages require an extra dose of motivation on your part.

The first thing you should do when you hit a plateau is to tell yourself, *I refused to become discouraged by this.* Discouragement is what leads to binges. This is why inspirational reading or motivational tapes are so important.

Second, you need to remind yourself, *There may be reasons for this—some of them I may need to check out.*

Weight-loss and fat-loss programs alike cause major adjustments to the body's chemistry. Sometimes fluids are retained, sometimes the shift from fat weight to muscle weight comes into play, and sometimes there are other problems. If the scales don't budge for a week. Use your body fat caliper. You are probably only gaining muscle weight, which is great.

Review how you have been eating and exercising. Have you been cheating? Have you cut your workouts short? Are you drinking enough water? Are you doing your cardiovascular exercises?

If you are doing the right things, remind yourself that good things are happening at the cellular level of your body. These processes are ones you can't see yet, but you will see them if you continue to do them!

Third, you need to say to yourself again and again, *Have a little patience!*

Most people who deal with learning and habit-building say that it takes three to four weeks for a new habit to be fully ingrained into a person's life. *Expect* to need three or four weeks of consciously and conscientiously *working* at building new habits.

Even after a new habit has been "installed" in the operating system of your own brain computer, you will need to periodically upgrade the system by refocusing on specifics of your new pattern of living. Overall, however, you likely will find that you don't have to think about some things anymore. You will just automatically do them and they will feel right to you. When you reach this point, congratulations! You have developed a life pattern you can live all your life!

ALWAYS REMEMBER . . .

This program works. I have proven it. It will work for you. Apply—and continue to apply—the twelve keys to this program and I guarantee that they will result in maximum fat loss!

CONCLUSION

The human body stores and loses weight in the same sequence. In other words, when the human body begins to store excess fat, it does so in an orderly way, proceeding from the abdominal area to the deep tissues surrounding the abdominal area, followed by the superficial areas around the body, then the buttocks, and lastly, the thighs and arms. When a person begins to lose fat, the order is the same: abdomen first, deep abdominal tissues, superficial areas all over the body, buttocks, thighs and arms.

"But," you may be saying to yourself, "what about 'spot-reducing?'" A wide variety of exercises, creams, and dietary supplements claim to help a person lose fat in isolated areas. The only true spot-reducing method available is liposuction, an invasive surgical procedure.

If you truly want to lose a problem-area of stored fat, stay with a low-glycemic diet, stay with your exercise program, and keep drinking pure water and taking your vitamin and mineral supplements. And . . . give yourself time!

BIBLIOGRAPHY

Adamo, M., D. LeRoith, J. Simon, J. Roth, et al. "Effect of Altered Nutritional States on Insulin Receptors." *Annual Review of Nutrition* 1988: 149–166.

Assman, G. and H. Schulte, "Relation of High- Density Lipoprotein Cholesterol and Triglycerides to Incidence of Atherosclerotic Coronary Artery Disease (The PROCAM Experience)." *American Journal of Cardiology* 70 (1992): 733–737.

Chen, Y. D., A. M. Coulston, M. Y. Zhou, et al. "Why Do Low-fat High-carbohydrate Diets Accentuate Postprandial Lipemia in Patients with NIDDM?" *Diabetes Care* 18(1) (1995): 10–16.

Faure, P., J. L. Lafond, C. Coudray, et al. "Zinc Prevents the Structural and Functional Properties of Free Radical Treated-insulin." *Biochimica et Biophysica Acta* 1209 (1994): 260–264.

Garg, A., J. Bantle, R. Henry, et al. "Effects of Varying Carbohydrate Content of Diet in Patients with Non-Insulin-Dependent Diabetes Mellitus." *Journal of the American Medical Association* 271 (1994): 1421–1428.

Jain, S. K., R. McVie, J. J. Jaramillo, et al. "Effect of modest vitamin E supplementation on blood glycated hemoglobin and triglyceride levels and red cell indices in type I diabetic patients." *Journal of American Col. Nutrition* 15(5) (1996): 458–461.

Laws, A., A. C. King, W. L. Haskell, and G. M. Reaven. "Relation of fasting plasma insulin concentration to high-density lipoprotein cholesterol and triglyceride concentration in men." *Arteriosclerosis Throm.* 11 (1991): 1636–1642.

Paolisso, G., S. Sgambato, and G. Pizza, et al. "Improved insulin response and action by chronic magnesium administration in aged NIDDM subjects." *Diabetes Care* 12 (1989): 265–269.

Reaven, G. M. "Pathophysiology of insulin resistance in human disease." *Physiological Reviews* 75(3) (1995): 473–485.

Reaven, G. M. "Role of insulin resistance in human disease." *Diabetes* 37 (1988): 1495-1507.

Tobey, T. A., M. Greenfield, F. Kraemer, and G. M. Reaven. "Relationship between insulin resistance, insulin secretion, very low-density lipoprotein kinetics and plasma triglyceride levels in normal triglyceridemic men." *Metabolism* 30 (1981): 165–171.

Zavaroni, I., P. Coruzzi, L. Bonini, et al. "Association between salt sensitivity and insulin con-centrations in patients with hypertension." *American Journal of Hypertension* 8 (1995): 855–858.

Zavaroni, I., L. Bonini, M. Fantuzzi, et al. "Hyperinsulinaemia, Obesity, and Syndrome X." *Journal of Internal Medicine* 235 (1994): 51–56.

Morbidity and Mortality Weekly Report 46 (1997): 1013–26.

Blundell, J. E. and A. H. Hill. "Paradoxical Effects of an Intense Sweetener (Aspartame) on Appetite." *Lancet* (1986): 1092–93.

Boehm, M. and J. Bada. "Racemization of aspartic acid and phenylalanine in the sweetener aspartame at 100 degrees C." *Proc. Natl. Acad. Sci.*, USA 81 (1984):

Garriga, M. and D. Metcalf. "Aspartame Intolerance." *Annals of Allergy* 61 (1988): 63–66.

Ishu, H. "Incidence of brain tumors in rats fed aspartame." *Toxicol Letters* 7 (1981): 433–37.

Saleman, M. "The morbidity and mortality of brain tumors." *Neurol. Clin.* 3 (1985): 229–57.

Monte, W. C. "Aspartame: Methanol and the Public Health." *Journal of Applied Nutrition* 16(1), abstract (1984):

Olney, J. W., et al. "Brain Damage in Mice from Voluntary Ingestion of Glutamate and Aspartame." *Neurobehavioral Toxicology* 2 (1980): 125–29.

Partridge, W. M. "Potential Effects of the Dipeptide Sweetener Aspartame on the Brain." *Nutrition and the Brain* 7 (1986): 199–241.

Ptenza, D., et al. "Aspartame: Clinical Update." *Connecticut Medical Journal* 53(7) (1989): 3997–3400.

Roberts, H. J. "Does Aspartame Cause Human Brain Cancer?" *Journal of Advancement in Medicine* 4(1) (1991): 231–40.

Roberts, H. J. Roberts. "Reactions attributed to aspartame-containing products: 551 cases." *Journal of Applied Nutrition* 49 (1988): 85–94.

"Sweet Suspicions." Three-part *CBS Nightly News* series. January 1984. Transcript reprinted in *Congressional Record.* S108–S126.

U.S. Air Force. "Aspartame Alert." *Flying Safety* 48(5) (1992): 20–21.

U.S. Department of Health and Human Services. National Institutes of Health. National Library of Medicine pamphlet. Current Bibliography series. *Adverse Effects of Aspartame—January '86 through December '90,* 1991. This report lists 167 citations of aspartame studies.

"Most Scientists in Poll Doubt NutraSweet's Safety." *New York Times.* 17 August 1987.

Walton, R. G., et al. "Adverse Reactions to Aspartame: Double-Blind Challenge in Patients with a Vulnerable Population." *Biological Psychiatry* 34 (1993): 13–17.

Wurtman, R. J. "Aspartame: possible effect on seizure susceptibility." *Lancet* 2 (1985): 1060.

R. G. "Seizure and mania after high intake of aspartame." *Psychopathology* 17 (1984): 98–106.

NOTES

INTRODUCTION

1. Michael Fumento, *The Fat of the Land: The Obesity Epidemic and What Overweight Americans Can Do About It* (New York: Viking, 1997).
2. Ibid.
3. Ibid.

CHAPTER 4

1. P. Benjamin and S. Lamp, *Understanding Sports Massage* (Champaign, IL: Human Kinetics, 1996),
2. S. Brownlee, "Coming to Our Senses," *U.S. News & World Report,* January 1997, 55-56.
3. M. Beck, *Milady's Theory and Practice of Therapeutic Massage* (Albany, NY: Milady Publishing Company, 1994)
4. My wife, Sharon, has an excellent cookbook that includes many good recipes as well as grocery-shopping and cooking tips. You can order this by calling our office: 1–800–726–1834.
5. My *Forever Fit* tape series or exercise videos can give you personal-trainer-style help: 1–800–726–1834.

CHAPTER 5

1. R. W. Bryner et al., "The Effects of Exercise Intensity on Body Composition, Weight Loss, and Dietary Composition in Women," *Journal of American Coll. Nutrition* 16 (1997): 68-73; A. Geliebter et al., "Effects of Strength or Aerobic Training on Body Composition, Resting Metabolic Rate, and Peak Oxygen Consumption in Obese Dieting Subjects," *American Journal of Clinical Nutrition* 66(3) (1997): 557–63; W. J. Kraemer et al., "Physiological Adaptations to a Weight-Loss Dietary Regimen and Exercise Programs in Women," *Journal of Applied Physiology* 83 (1997): 270–279.
2. N. L. Keim et al., "Weight Loss Is Greater with Consumption of Large Morning Meals and Fat Mass Is Preserved with Large Evening Meals in Women on a Controlled Weight Reduction Regimen," *Journal of Nutrition* 127 (1997): 75–82; R. B. Kreider et al., *Overtraining in Sport* (Champaign, IL: Human Kinetics Publishers, 1998)

3. V. Van Harmelen et al., "Mechanisms Involved in the Regulation of Free Fatty Acid Release from Isolated Human Fat Cells by Acylation-stimulating Protein and Insulin," *Journal of Biological Chemistry* 274(26) (1999): 18243–51.

4. C. Simon et al., "Twenty-four-hour Rhythms of Plasma Glucose and Insulin Secretion Rate in Regular Night Workers," *American Journal of Physiological Endocrinol Metabolism* 274(3) (2000): E413–20.

5. David J. A. Jenkins et al., "Glycemic Index of Foods: A Physiological Basis for Carbohydrate Exchange," *The American Journal of Clinical Nutrition* 34 (1981): 362–66.

6. M. Varnier et al., "Stimulatory Effect of Glutamine on Glycogen Accumulation in Human Skeletal Muscle," *American Journal of Physiology* 269(2) E309–15; S. Maehlum et al., "Splanchnic Glucose and Muscle Glycogen Metabolism after Glucose Feeding During Postexercise Recovery," *American Journal of Physiology* 235(3) (1978): E255–60.

CHAPTER 6

1. M. Piatti et al., "Hypocaloric High-Protein Diet Improves Glucose Oxidation and Spares Lean Body Mass: Comparison to Hypocaloric High-Carbohydrate Diet," *Metabolism* 43 (1994): 1481–87.

2. G. Boumous and P. Gold, "The Biological Activity of Undernatured Dietary Whey Proteins: Role of Glutathione," *Clinical Investigative Medicine* 14:4 (1991): 296-309; G. Boumous and P. L. Kongshavn, "Differential Effect of Dietary Protein Type on the B Cell and T Cell Immune Responses in Mice," *Journal of Nutrition* 115(1)1 (1985): 1403–04; P. F. Fox, *Developments in Dairy Chemistry Proteins* (London: Elsevier Applied Science Publishing, 1982, 1989), 1–4.

3. V. Akiba and L. S. Jensen, "Temporal Effect of Change in Diet Composition on Plasma Estradiol and Thyroxine Concentrations and Hepatic Lipogenesis in Laying Hens" *Journal of Nutrition* 113(10) (1983): 2178–84; J. W. Anderson et al., "Meta Analysis of the Effects of Soy Protein Intake on Serum Lipids," *New England Journal of Medicine* 333 (1995): 276–82; C. A. Barth et al., "Difference of Plasma Amino Acids Following Casein or Soy Protein Intake: Significance for Differences of Serum Lipid Concentrations," *Journal of Nutritional Science Vitaminology* 36 (supplement II) (1990): S111–17; C. A. Barth and M. Pfeuffer, "Dietary Protein and Atherogenesis," *Klin. Wochenschr.* 66(4) (1988): 135–43.

4. J. Cosnes et al., "Improvement in Protein Absorption with a Small Peptide-Based Diet in Patients with High Jejunostomy," *Nutrition* 8(6) (1992): 406–11; G. K. Grimble et al., "Effect of Peptide Chain Length on Amino Acid and Nitrogen Absorption from Two Lactalbumin Hydrolysates in the Normal Human Jejunum," *Clinical Science* 71(1) (1986): 65-69.

CHAPTER 7

1. N. L. Keim et al., "Weight Loss Is Greater with Consumption of Large Morning Meals and Fat-Free Mass Is Preserved with Large Evening Meals in Women on a Controlled

Weight Reduction Regimen," *Journal of Nutrition* 127 (1997): 75–82; R. B. Kreider et al., *Overtraining in Sport* (Champaign, IL: Human Kinetics Publishers, 1998),

2. J. B. Miller, E. Pang, and L. Bramall, "Rice: A High or Low Glycemic Index Food?" *American Journal of Clinical Nutrition* 56 (1992): 1034–36.

CHAPTER 8

1. USCA CSFII Survey

2. *Agricultural Research,* June 2000: 17.

3. J. P. Burke et al., "Rapid rise in the Incidence of Type 2 Diabetes from 1987 to 1996," *Arch. Internal Medicine* 159 (1999): 1450–56.

4. A growing number of studies are related to Syndrome X. Please see the bibliography for a list of some of the many research studies that support the conclusions presented in this book.

CHAPTER 9

1. Hans-Heinrich Reckeweg, M.D., "The Adverse Influence of Pork Consumption on Health," *Biological Therapy,* 1(2) (1983):

2. The National Academy of Sciences, *Nutrition, Diet, and Cancer,* 1982.

3. Sandra Steingraber, Ph.D., *Living Downstream: A Scientist's Personal Investigation of Cancer and the Environment* (New York: Vintage Books, 1997), 132-134.

4. Steingraber, *Living Downstream,* 142.

5. News release issued in 1999 by Mike Ostasz, Division of Environmental Health, Alaska Department of Environmental Conservation, 555 Cordova Street, Anchorage, AK 99501-2617.

6. See the official Centers for Disease Control (CDC) warning notice posted on the U.S. Government's official CDC web site at http://www.cdc.gov/ncidod/diseases/food-born/vi briov u.htm

7. Sharon Broer's *Eat, Drink and Be Healthy Cookbook* can be ordered from our office: 1–800–726-1834.

8. I recommend the book *Exitotoxins—The Taste that Kills* by Russell Blaylock.

9. Dean Ornish, M.D., *Eat More, Weigh Less* (New York: HarperCollins, 1993), 34.

10. John A. McDougall, M.D., and Mary A. McDougall, *The McDougall Plan* (Piscataway, NJ: New Century Publishers, 1983), 5.

11. S. Bahna, *Allergies to Milk* (New York: Grune and Stratton, 1980)

12. For more information on goat's milk and children's diets, I recommend my wife's book *Train Up Your Children in the Way They Should Eat.* You can order a copy from our office: 1–800–726-1834.

13. H. B. Fu et al., "Dietary Fat Intake and the Risk of Coronary Heart Disease in Women" (abstract), *New England Journal of Medicine,* 227(21) (1997): 1491–99; M. W. Gillman et al., "Margarine Intake and Subsequent Coronary Heart Disease in Men," *Epidemiology,* 8(2) (1997): 144–49; L. Kohlmeier et al., "Adipose Tissue Trans Fatty Acids and Breast Cancer in the European Community Multicenter Study on Antioxidants, Myocardial Infarction, and Breast Cancer," *Cancer Epidemiology, Biomarkers & Prevention,* 6(9) (1997): 705-710.

CHAPTER 10

1. The best green product I have found is called "Green Life." It is available through my office: 1–800–726–1834.

CHAPTER 12

1. Sandra Steingraber, *Living Downstream: A Scientist's Personal Investigation of Cancer and the Environment* (New York: Vintage Books, 1997), 96–97.

2. Fred Van Lue, founder, WaterWise Inc., "Water: Why You Absorb As Many Toxins in One Hot Shower As If You Had Drunk Eight Glasses of Contaminated Water," interview in *Forever Fit at 20, 30, 40 & Beyond,*

3. You can call my office for more information about water filtration systems: 1–800–726–1834.

4. I address this topic thoroughly in my book *Maximum Energy,* which can be ordered through my office: 1-800-726-1834.

5. A. Neims and R. von Borstel, "Caffeine: Metabolism and Biochemical Mechanisms of Actions," *Nutrition and the Brain,* vol. 2, eds. R. Wurtman and J. Wurtman (New York: Raven Press, 1983) P. Brooks, "Measuring the Effect of Caffeine Restriction on Fibrocystic Breast Disease," *Journal of Rep. Medicine,* 26 (1981): 279.

6. Dean Ornish, M.D., *Eat More, Weigh Less* (New York: HarperCollins, 1993), 39.

7. P. M. Suter, Y. Schutz, and E. Jequier, "The Effect of Ethanol on Fat Storage in Healthy Subjects," *New England Journal of Medicine,* 326(15) (1982): 983–7.

CHAPTER 13

1. D. Thomas-Dobersen, "Calculation of Aspartame Intake in Children," *Journal of the American Dietetic Association* 89(6) (1989): 831–33; Federal Register 44 (1979): 31716–18.

2. Pre-approval FDE study "E70," Olney, 1987, 7.

3. For more information about aspartame, see the list of related literature in the bibliography. I have also prepared my own in-depth report on aspartame, which is available through my office: 1-800-226-1834.

4. L. Bonvie, B. Bonvie, and D. Gates, *The Stevia Story* (Atlanta, GA: B.E.D., 1997), 38.

CHAPTER 14

1. V. E. Iron, interview, *Healthview Newsletter* 1 (1983):

2. If you have high blood pressure or high cholesterol, I recommend my *Eat, Drink, and Be Healthy* program, which is available through my office: 1–800–726–1834.

3. D. Y. Graham et al., "The Effect of Bran on Bowel Function in Constipation," *American Journal of Gastroenterology* 77 (1982): 599–603.

4. The only chemical laxative I recommend to my clients—which works well and is not addictive—is Atru Aloe. The bulk laxative product I carry for sale is a mixture of different fibers. You can call my office for details: 1–800–726–1834.

5. D. S. Gray, "The Clinical Uses of Dietary Fiber," *American Family Physician,* 92(5) (February 1995): 419–26.

6. H. Philipson, "Dietary Fiber in the Diabetic Diet," *Accta Med Scan* (supplement) 671 (1983): 91–93; T. Poynard et al., "Reduction of Post-Prandial Insulin Needs by Pectin

as Assessed by the Artificial Pancreas in Insulin-Dependent Diabetics," *Diabetes & Metabolism,* 8(3) (1982): 187–89.

7. M. L. Burr et al., "Dietary Fiber, Blood Pressure and Plasma Cholesterol," *Nutritional Research* 5 (1985): 465–472; J. Anderson, "Plant Fiber and Blood Pressure," *Annals of Internal Medicine,* 98 (1983): 842.

8. On the seven-day cleansing program I recommend to my clients, I provide concentrated nutrients to help prevent protein catabolism. I also believe a person should never fast more than one day without the use of colonics, which can be done in the privacy of your own home.

CHAPTER 15

1. P. Glasziou et al., "Managing the Overweight and Obese: A Low Fat Approach," *Aust. Family Physician* 26 (1997): 1259–63; M. L. Klem et al., "A Descriptive Study of Individuals Successful at Long-Term Maintenance of Substantial Weight Loss," *American Journal of Clinical Nutrition* 66 (1997): 239–46; W. C. Miller et al., "A Meta-Analysis of the Past 25 Years of Weight Loss Research Using Diet, Exercise or Diet Plus Exercise Intervention," *Int. J. Obes. Relat. Metab. Disord.* 21 (1997): 941–47.

2. U. Erasmus, *Fats That Heal, Fats That Kill* (Burnaby, British Columbia, Canada: Alive Books, 1993),

3. U. Erasmus, *Fats that Heal, Fats that Kill,*

4. J. Budwig, *Flax Oil as a True Aid Against Arthritis, Heart Infarction, Cancer and Other Diseases* (Vancouver, British Columbia, Canada: Apple Publishing Company, 1959, 1994),

CHAPTER 16

1. I have both men's and women's exercise videos—for beginning, intermediate, and advanced exercise, including an exercise video for those who are professional athletes. The videos covers the do's and don'ts of exercise in great detail. Call my office for more information: 1-800-726-1834.

2. R. W. Bryner et al., "The Effects of Exercise Intensity on Body Composition, Weight Loss, and Dietary Composition in Women," *Journal of American Coll. Nutrition* 16 (1997): 68–73; H. E. Carmichael et al., "Lower Fat Intake as a Predictor of Initial and Sustained Weight Loss in Obese Subjects Consuming an Otherwise Ad Libitum Diet," *Journal of the American Dietetic Association* 98(1) (1998): 45–49; P. Glasziou et al., "Managing the Overweight and Obese: A Low Fat Approach," *Aust. Fam. Physician* 26 (1997): 1259–63; M. L. Klem et al., "A Descriptive Study of Individuals Successful at Long-Term Maintenance of Substantial Weight Loss," *American Journal of Clinical Nutrition* 66 (1997): 239–46; D. West and B. York, "Dietary Fat, Genetic Predisposition, and Obesity: Lessons from Animal Models," *American Journal of Clinical Nutrition* 67 (1998): 505S–12S.

3. A. Geliebter et al., "Effects of Strength or Aerobic Training on Body Composition, Resting Metabolic Rate, and Peak Oxygen Consumption in Obese Dieting Subjects," *American Journal of Clinical Nutrition* 66(3) (1997): 557–63; W. J. Kraemer et al., "Physiological Adaptations to a Weight-Loss Dietary Regimen and Exercise Programs in Women," *Journal of Applied Physiology* 83 (1997): 270–79; W. C. Miller et al., "A

Meta-Analysis of the Past 25 Years of Weight Loss Research Using Diet, Exercise or Diet Plus Exercise Intervention," *Int. J. Obes. Relat. Metab. Disord.* 21 (1997): 941–47; C. Melby et al., "Effect of Acute Resistance Exercise on Postexercise Energy Expenditure and Resting Metabolic Rate," *Journal of Applied Physiology* 75(4) (1993): 1847–53.

4. We have a great selection of audio tapes available through my office: 1–800–726–1834.

CHAPTER 17

1. W. W. Campbell and R. A. Anderson, "Effects of Aerobic Exercise and Training on the Trace Minerals Chromium, Zinc and Copper," *Sports Medicine* 4(1) (1987): 9–18; A. Singh et al., "Biochemical Indices of Selected Trace Minerals in Men: Effect of Stress," *American Journal of Clinical Nutrition* 53(1) (1991): 126–31; A. Singh et al., "Magnesium, Zinc, and Copper Status of U.S. Navy SEAL Trainees," *American Journal of Clinical Nutrition* 49(4) (1989): 695–700; L. M. Weight et al., "Vitamin and Mineral Status of Trained Athletes Including the Effects of Supplementation," *American Journal of Clinical Nutrition* 47(2) (1988): 186–91.

2. Theis study was published in the *American Journal of Clinical Nutrition* in 1993

3. For hair analysis information, call my office: 1-800-726-1834.

4. If you have difficulty finding any of these supplements, or have additional questions about them, feel free to call my office: 1–800–726–1834.

5. R. A. Anderson, "Effects of Chromium on Body Composition and Weight Loss," *Nutritional Review* 56(9) (1998): 266–70.

6. R. A. Anderson et al., "Effects of Supplemental Chromium on Patients with Symptoms of Reactive Hypoglycemia," *Metabolism* 36(4) (1987): 351–55.

7. R. A. Anderson et al., "Effects of Exercise (Running) on Serum Glucose, Insulin, Glucagon, and Chromium Excretion," *Diabetes* 31(3) (1982): 212–16; S. Davies et al., "Age-Related Decreases in Chromium Levels in 51,665 Hair, Sweat, and Serum Samples from 40,872 Patients—Implications for the Prevention of Cardiovascular Disease and Type II Diabetes Mellitus," *Metabolism* 46(5) (1997): 469–73.

8. D. C. Nieman, "Exercise, Infection, and Immunity," *International Journal of Sports Medicine* 15(S3) (1994): S131–41; E. Roth et al., "Glutamine: An Anabolic Effector" *Journal of Parent. Ent. Nutrition* 14 (1990): 1305–65.

9. P. J. Collip et al., "Zinc Deficiency: Improvement in Growth and Growth Hormone Levels with Oral Zinc Therapy," *Ann. Nutr. Metab.* 26(5) (1982): 287–90.

10. R. K. Chandra, "Excessive Intake of Zinc Impairs Immune Responses," *Journal of the American Medical Association* 252(1) (1984): 1443–46.

11. Informative reports on high blood pressure, diabetes, depression, cancer, and impotency are covered in my *Eat, Drink & Be Healthy* program. If you are interested, call my office: 1–800–726–1834.

12. L. R. Brilla and T. F. Haley, "Effect of Magnesium Supplemen-tation on Strength Training in Humans," *Journal of American Coll. Nutrition* 11:3 (1992): 326–29.

13. S. S. Natah et al., "Metabolic Response to Lactitol and Xylitol in Healthy Men," *American Journal of Clinical Nutrition* 65(1) (1997): 947–50.

14. P. J. Arciero et al., "Effects of Creatine Supplementation and Weight Training on

Resting Metabolic Rate and 1RM in College-Aged Males," *International Sport Nutrition Conference,* 1997.

15. We carry the best calcium supplement on the market through our office. Call me if you want more information: 1–800–726–1834.

16. R. Pasquali et al., "Effects of Chronic Administration of Ephedrine During Very Low Calorie Diets on Energy Expenditure, Protein Metabolism and Hormone Levels in Obese Subjects." *Clinical Science* 82(1) (1992): 85–92; B. Buemann et al., "The Effect of Ephedrine Plus Caffeine on Plasma Lipids and Lipoproteins During a 4.2 Mg/day Diet," *International Journal of Obesity* 18 (1994): 329–32; M. R. Wooten et al., "Intracerebral Hemorrhage and Vasculitis Related to Ephedrine Abuse," *Annals of Neurology* 33 (1983): 337–40.

17. M. Berlan et al., "Plasma Catecholamine Levels and Lipid Mobilization Induced by Yohimbine in Obese and Non-Obese Women," *Int. Journal of Obes.* 15(5) (1991): 305–15; D. Muller-Wieland et al., "Inhibition of Fatty Acid Synthesis by Stimulation of Alpha- and Beta-Adrenergic Receptors in Human Mononuclear Leukocytes," *Horm. Metab. Res.* 26(4) (1994): 169–72.

18. R. T. Stanko, H. R. Reynolds, R. Houson, J. E. Janosky, and R. Wolf, "Pyruvate Supplementation of a Low-Cholesterol, Low-Fat Diet: Effects on Plasma Lipid Concentrations and Body Composition in Hyperlipidemic Patients," *American Journal of Clinical Nutrition* 59(2) (1994): 423–27; R. T. Stanko, H. R. Reynolds, K. D. Lonchar, and J. E. Arch, "Plasma Lipid Concentrations in Hyperlipidemic Patients Consuming a High-Fat Diet Supplemented with Pyruvate for 6 Weeks," *American Journal of Clinical Nutrition* 56(5) (1992): 950–54; R. T. Stanko, D. L. Tietze, and J. E. Arch, "Body Composition, Energy Utilization, and Nitrogen Metabolism with a Severely Restricted Diet Supplemented with Dihydroxyacetone and Pyruvate," *American Journal of Clinical Nutrition* 55(4) (1992): 771–76; R. T. Tanko, D. L. Tietze, and J. E. Arch, "Body Composition, Energy Utilization, and Nitrogen Metabolism with a 4.25–MJ/d Low-Energy Diet Supplemented with Pyruvate," *American Journal of Clinical Nutrition* 56(4) (1992): 630–35.

19. G. Sjodin et al., "Biochemical Mechanisms for Oxygen Free Radical Formation During Exercise," *Sports Medicine* 10(4) (1990): 236–54.

20. R. Klatz, M.D., *Grow Young with HGH* (New York, HarperCollins, 1997),

21. D. Rudman et al, "Effects of Human Growth Hormone in Men Over 60 Years Old," *New England Journal of Medicine* 323 (1990): 1–5; D. Rudman et al., "Effects of Human Growth Hormone on Body Composition in Elderly Men," *Horm. Res.* 36 (Supplement 1) (1991): 73–81.

CHAPTER 18

1. C. Scherwitz and O. Braun-Falco, "So-called Cellulite," *Journal of Dermatol. Surg. Oncol.* 4 (1978): 230–34.

2. F. Nurnberger and O. Muller, "So-called Cellulite: An Invented Disease," *J. Dermatol. Surg. Oncol.* 4 (1978): 221–29.

3. F. Nurnberger et al., " Behundlungsergebnisse Bei der Sog. 'Cellulitis' Mit Verteilerenzymen im Einfachen Blindversuch," *Arch. Dermatol. Forsch.* 29 (1972): 173–81.

4. F. Nurnberger et al., Behundlungsergebnisse Bei der Sog. 'Cellulitis' Mit Verteilerenzymen im Einfachen Blindversuch," *Arch. Dermatol. Forsch.* 29 (1972): 173–81; F. Nurnberger and B. Schroter: "Behundlungsergebnisse Bei der Sog. Zellulitis Mit Verteilerenzymen im Doppelblindversuch," *A. Hautkr.* 48 (1973): 1009–17. These studies specifically tested thiomucase, nemectron, and alec eden-slenderetone treatments.
5. Monograph: Centella asiatica, Indena S.p.A., Milan, Italy, 1987.
6. F. Aichinger et al., "Neue befunde zur pharmakodynamik von bioflavoiden und das Rosskastanien Saponine Aescin als Grundlage Ihrer Anwendung in der Therapie," *Arzniem Forsch* 14 (1964): 892.
7. Monograph: Bladderwrack, Indena S.p.A., Milan, Italy, 1987.

CHAPTER 19
1. As quoted in a Newsweek, Inc. 2000 news feature posted on the internet.
2. My wife, Sharon, has written a book titled *Train Up Your Children in the Way They Should Eat,* which is available through my office: 1-800-726-1834.

CHAPTER 20
1. "Rationale for the surgical treatment of severe obesity" (American Society for Bariatric Surgery, Gainesville, FL, 1997). Retrieved June 10, 1998, from http://www.asbs.org/html /ration.html#NONOP.
2. "Side effects of the gastric bypass and the gastric banding" (Alvarado Center for Surgical Weight Control, 1997). Retrieved June 10, 1998, from http://www. gastricbypass.com
3. Center for the surgical treatment of obesity (1996) Retrieved June 10, 1998, from http://www.cstobesity.com/patient,htm
4. Miller Fahey, "Management of the overweight patient" *Family Practice Recertification* 19(8) (1997): 45-74.
5. F. Greenway, "Surgery for Obesity," *Endocrinology and Metabolism Clinics* 25(4) (1996):
6. "Treating severe obesity" (Mayo Health Clinic, 1997). Retrieved June 10, 1998, from
7. "Gastrip Surgery for Severe Obesity" (National Institute of Diabetes and Digestive and Kidney Disease, Bethesda, MD, 1998). Retrieved June 10, 1998, from http://www.niddk.nih.gov/ Gastric/Gastsurg.html.
8. National Institute of Health Technology Assessment Conference Panel, "Methods of voluntary weight loss and control" *Annals of Internal Medicine* 116(8)(1992): 942-949.
9. "Gastrointestinal Surgery for Severe Obesity (National Institute of Health, 1991 Consensus Statement). Retrieved June 10, 1998, from gopher://gopher.nih.gov:70/ 00/clin/cdcs/individual/84.obs
10. "Maximizing your chances of getting an insurance approval the first time" (Obesity Law & Advocacy Center, San Diego, CA, 1998). Retrieved June 10, 1998, from http://www.obesitylaw.com/maximize.htm
11. Rarh et al, "Primary Care Management of Adult Obesity" *Physician Assistant Journal,* 22(4): 35-56.

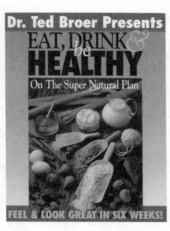

EAT, DRINK, AND BE HEALTHY TAPE PROGRAM
by Dr. Ted and Sharon Broer
Our six week program to optimal Health and Energy!

Tape 1: The Top Ten Foods Never to Eat

Tape 2: Forever Slim (Do's and Don'ts of Weight Loss)

Tape 3: Winning Choices for Your Health

Tape 4: Double Your Energy, Double Your Output

Tape 5: Simplifying the Supermarket Safari

Tape 6: Foods That Heal

Tape 7: Food Choices: Facts & Myths

Tape 8: Answers to Our Most Frequently Asked Questions.

Plus reports on: ADD, Hypertension, Cancer, Diabetes, Depression, and Prostate Problems.

FOREVER FIT: AT 20, 30, 40, AND BEYOND TAPE SERIES
by Dr. Ted Broer
Lose Weight* Feel Great* Fitness/Health Series
Our latest, up-to-date series on Health, Nutrition, Sports Medicine, and exercise!

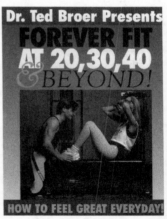

Tape 1: Fat Loss, Not Weight Loss—The Key to Looking Great! Hormones and How They Control the Body.

Tape 2: Exercise—Its Role in Burning Fat/Lean Muscle Mass—What Types & How much

Tape 3: Trace Minerals, Vitamin Supplements, Fatty Acids/Join Repair and Arthritis

Tape 4: Artificial Sweeteners/Chemicals and Foods in Our Environment to Avoid

Tape 5: Chronic Fatigue Syndrome, Yeast Infection, Hypoglycemia, and Your Immune System

Tape 6: Constipation, the Colon, and Your Health

Tape 7: Fasting: The Physical & Spiritual Benefits

Tape 8: Water: Use a Filter or Be a Filter/Why You Absorb As Many Toxins in One Hot Shower as If You Had Drunk 8 Glasses of Contaminated Water.

Plus reports on: Nutrasweet, Constipation, Eating for body fat loss, Yeast infections, Epstein-Barr, and Chronic Fatigue Syndrome

TO ORDER CALL 1-800-726-1834

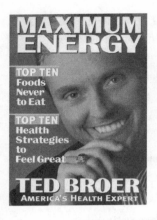

MAXIMUM ENERGY BOOK
by Dr. Ted Broer

- The Top Ten Foods Never to Eat!
- The Top Ten Health Strategies for Maximum Energy!
- Double your energy in 30 days with the right choices in this insightful book!

MAXIMUM ENERGY COOKBOOK
by Sharon Broer

A Health Guide to Survive! This book is an ideal gift for loved ones.
It includes:

- Back to basics recipes
- Infant, toddler, & children's diet
- Holiday Recipes
- Drinks, shakes, and coolers
- Fruit, vegetables, grains, and meat recipes
- Stress avoidance, exercise, water, goat's milk, and more . . .

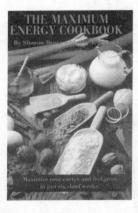

TRAIN UP YOUR CHILDREN IN THE WAY THEY SHOULD EAT
The Ultimate childrens program
A must for every concerned parent
by Sharon Broer

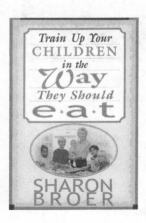

- Ensure the good health of your unborn baby.
- Nourish the infant and toddler so they can thrive.
- Protect and enhance the all-important immune systems of your children.
- Fuel active minds and bodies for complete physical and mental growth.
- Learn what your pediatrician won't tell you about nutrition and your child's health
- Stop serving the beverage that's more toxic than lead!
- No Ritalin
- No Ear infection
- No Allergies

TO ORDER CALL 1-800-726-1834

EAT, DRINK AND BE HEALTHY EXERCISE VIDEOS

by Dr. Broer

A scientific Approach to Athletic Conditioning and Proper Nutrition.
It Includes:

- Non Impact Training
- Lean Muscle Growth & Fat Loss in 6 Weeks
- For Men and Women of all ages
- Three tape series for Men or Women - 6 total tapes
- Lifetime warranty on videos

UNDERSTANDING GOD'S DIETARY PRINCIPLES TAPE SERIES

This one answers all the Biblical Nutrition Questions
by Dr. Broer

Tape 1: How God's Dietary Principles Relate to Us

Tape 2: In Depth Scriptural Overview

Tape 3: How to Break the Dietary Curses of Degenerative Disease

HYPOGLYCEMIA: A SENSIBLE APPROACH TAPE SERIES

by Dr. Broer

Tape 1: Sugar & Controlling Hypoglycemia

Tape 2: Sugar and the American Sweet Tooth

Tape 3: What has Happened to Our Health?

If you have it, you need this series.

NUTRITION AND YOUR HEALTHY HEART TAPE SERIES

by Dr. Broer

Tape 1: Preventing Heart Disease

Tape 2: Exercising the Smart Way

Tape 3: Stress and Your Health

Learn how to keep this critical organ in top shape.

NATURAL COOKING FOR THE HOLIDAYS TAPE SERIES

by Sharon Broer

Tape 1: Using Meat Replacements and Grains

Tape 2: Holiday Meal Planning

Tape 3: Sugar Replacements and Holiday Desserts

For those who ask: "Where do I start?"

BREAKING THE DIETARY CURSES OF CANCER TAPE SERIES

by Dr. Broer

Tape 1: Cancer Prevention

Tape 2: The Benefits of Fasting

Tape 3: Fiber and a Healthy Colon

Tape 4: God's Dietary Principles

Tape 5: Clean & Unclean Foods

The nation's 2nd largest killer can be prevented.

HELPING YOUR FAMILY MAKE DIETARY CHANGES TAPE SERIES

by Dr. Ted and Sharon Broer

Tape 1: Fiber & Food Preparation

Tape 2: Healthy Food Substitutes

Tape 3: Attitudes on Nutrition

This one makes it easy!

PREVENTING ARTHRITIS AND OSTEOPOROSIS TAPE SERIES

by Dr. Broer

Tape 1: Arthritis and Osteoporosis

Tape 2: The Importance of Calcium

Tape 3: Is Supplementation Necessary?

It's easier to prevent!

TRAIN UP A CHILD IN THE WAY HE SHOULD EAT TAPE SERIES

by Sharon Broer

Tape 1: Prenatal Nutrition

Tape 2: Infant & Toddler Nutrition

Tape 3: A Child's Diet

A must for those with children.